PORT IN THE
STORM

PORT IN THE
STORM

How to Make a Medical Decision and Live to Tell About It

Cole A. Giller, M.D., Ph.D.

LifeLine
Press®

A Regnery Publishing Company, Washington, D.C.

Library of Congress Cataloging-in-Publication Data

Giller, Cole A., 1954-
    How to make a medical decision (and live to tell about it) : a
    practical guide for those facing medical decisions for themselves or
    their loved ones / Cole A. Giller.
        p. cm.
    Includes bibliographical references and index.
        ISBN 0-89526-132-4
        1. Health--Decision making--Popular works. 2. Medicine--Decision
    making--Popular works. I. Title.
        RA776.95.G54 2003
        613--dc22
                                            2003017839

Published in the United States by
LifeLine Press
A Regnery Publishing Company
One Massachusetts Avenue, N.W.
Washington, DC 20001

Visit us at www.lifelinepress.com

Distributed to the trade by
National Book Network
4501 Forbes Boulevard, Suite 200
Lanham, MD 20706

Printed on acid-free paper

Manufactured in the United States of America

10 9 8 7 6 5 4 3 2 1

Books are available in quantity for promotional or premium use.
Write to Director of Special Sales, Regnery Publishing, Inc.,
One Massachusetts Avenue, N.W., Washington, DC 20001,
for information on discounts and terms or call (202) 216-0600.

The characters in this book are based on real people. The names and details have been altered to protect privacy.

The information contained in this book is not a substitute for medical counseling and care. All matters pertaining to your physical health should be supervised by a health care professional.

CONTENTS

Preface

Every Wednesday for the past twelve years I have spent my entire day helping other people make decisions that determine whether they will live or die. I am a neurosurgeon, and despite my training and commitment to the act of surgery, the most important thing I do for my patients is to help them decide how best to treat their neurological disease. And so each Wednesday I discuss with my patients whether to operate on their brain tumor, or whether to subject them to radiation therapy, or whether they wish to be treated at all. Even though these discussions are not physically demanding, by the end of the day I am bone-tired.

It is my job to present the options and the facts. What are the different operations, their pros and cons, and how often do they succeed? What are the risks of complications? And it is my patients' job to choose the options that make most sense for them. You would think that this is a straightforward process for us both; just list all the options and choose the best one.

But of course, important medical decisions are never straightforward. They are gut-wrenching puzzles for which most of us are poorly prepared, sprung upon us suddenly by the cruel accident that made us ill to begin with. They are made painfully complex by our changing attitudes towards doctors, the sheer mass of medical information that no one person can master, and the widespread availability of medical information on the Internet. And we try to soak up all this new information to give ourselves a do-it-yourself boost, hoping our new knowledge will propel us towards the correct medical decision. But effective decision making is an art requiring time, practice, and a trusted mentor, all in short supply when we are ill. Somehow, despite amazing medical advances, we can find ourselves left alone with our decisions and our stacks of computer printouts.

The importance of decision making has not been ignored by other fields. Business schools teach the science of decisions designed to enhance profits, and political scientists have brought decision scenarios to the fine art needed to cope with the dangers of nuclear weapons. A whole field of practical decision making emerged in the past two decades from our social psychologists, categorizing the mistakes we make, in order to improve decisions of all types. Doctors have devoted entire journals to the problem of decisions concerning public health. But scant attention has been paid to our personal decisions, especially the decision problems of those facing their own medical problems. There is little to guide us through the emotional and mental landscape of our tough medical decisions, and almost nothing has been written to teach us to apply what has been learned in these other fields.

My purpose here is to provide a handbook for those facing difficult medical decisions, believing as I do that in order to make good medical decisions, we must do far more than simply gather medical information. That is only the beginning. Decision making must include taking stock of our emotions and fears, constructing safe places for ourselves to think, interpreting medical information that makes sense to our own unique set of beliefs, and coming to conclusions that are meaningful and useful for our particular set of circumstances. And modern decision making should exploit the new discoveries made by our social psychologists and should use our doctors in ways never seen before. Yes, I will show you efficient strategies for extracting top-quality medical information from all possible sources, including the Internet. But the making of medical decisions is a complex art form, demanding a blend of human concerns and modern infomatics. My hope is that you will find both in a useful form within this handbook.

This book is divided into seven parts. In Part I, we discuss the current crisis in medical decisions, and how changes in our society and in ourselves have combined to obscure and complicate the decision process. We will then focus on the isolation and disorientation that arise naturally from our medical problems, and ways we can make this less painful as we consider our medical options. Part I also lays the mental groundwork for our plan to arrive at good medical decisions. Here we suggest certain attitudes about medical problems that will provide a mental and emotional basis for our later work in the decision-making process.

Part II introduces our six-step plan for medical decision making. Each step is outlined here in broad terms, then addressed in detail in individual chapters. Here you will find the nuts and bolts of medical decision making, everything from specific tips for using the Internet to suggestions for incorporating your personal beliefs and systems of meaning into the decision process.

Part III is devoted to the topic of your doctors: how to use them and how to interpret what they say. Here we look at our ambivalence in regard to doctors in ways rarely considered before, and discuss what to do if your doctors disagree.

In Part IV we look at the problems arising when we are making medical decisions for someone else, including the thorny problem of deciding for children.

In Part V we consider some special problems and pitfalls. Included are financial and money matters, indecision, and a variety of other special situations.

Part VI addresses what happens after you make your decision. We will discuss what makes a medical decision good, how to think about changing your mind, and offer some thoughts to consider when things go either well or poorly.

In Part VII we put it all together by demonstrating how you might make decisions if you have cancer. Even if you do not have cancer, this discussion will illustrate many decision-making principles that apply to other medical problems.

Acknowledgments

There are many people I want to thank for many things. First thanks go to my patients, who so generously taught me so much about the trials and agonies of medical decisions. Thanks also to the many medical mentors of my career (and you know who you are) for teaching me what it means to be responsible for a patient. Thanks to my parents, Donald and Benita Giller, for their encouragement and comments on the early manuscript. Thanks to Dr. Arlynn Mulne for her insightful help with the discussion about medical decisions for children. Thanks also go to Laura Berey for her support, enthusiasm, and comments, and to Dr. Duke Samson, Dr. Tom and Sandy Psarros, Nancy Diepenbrock, and Carol Crosby for their advice and critical review. And thanks to Bill Gilliland for his gentle encouragement and support.

Special thanks go to my agent, Laurie Harper, for believing in me and the book and for cajoling me to take correct paths. And I am likewise indebted to my editor, Molly Mullen, and LifeLine Press for their commitment to this book and for their professional skill and the energy they devoted to its fruition.

Finally and importantly, thanks to my children, Amelia, Claire, Charlie, and Megan, for putting up with Dad while he was writing, and thanks to my wife, Angie, for her optimism, insight, patience, and love that were so necessary for the creation of this book.

Why Read This Book?

This book is for you if you or your loved ones are facing a medical problem or a medical decision. And this book is for you if you think you might ever face a medical decision in the future.

Read this book because it is the only book that attends to every aspect of making medical decisions, the only book that takes you on a practical tour covering all the bases you need. Yes, medical decisions require efficient strategies to find medical information, and I will show you those here. But you also need a way to quickly evaluate these data, and a way to blend them with your own personal preferences and beliefs, a way that leads to decisions that are comfortable and meaningful to you. This book will help you do just that—it is the complete field handbook for anyone facing a medical decision.

You may be actively struggling with a medical decision for yourself or your loved ones. This book will give you valuable tips, strategies, and philosophies to guide you through this uncomfortable territory. You may have already made your decision, or you may be facing a medical problem that appears to have only a single choice. This book will help you reexamine decisions if needed, and will reinforce your comfort and confidence in the choices you have made. Or, you may simply be interested in a task that has always confronted human beings and that will continue to demand their attention for all time: that of making a medical decision for yourself or your loved ones.

So, this book is for you if the lonely and delicate task of making a medical decision ever has or ever will touch your life.

"In 1953 she was diagnosed with ovarian cancer. The family kept it a secret from her and their friends. She became progressively sicker and was never told what she had. Even the doctor did not tell her the truth. She never knew—although she probably suspected—until she died. She couldn't discuss it with anyone, and when she asked about her condition she was told that she would recover.

This was typical of those days."

—Benita Giller

Part I
Basics

The Decision Crisis

It is **1955,** and you have just learned that you have cancer. Your doctor tells you that surgery is the best treatment, and you gratefully agree. As they wheel you to the operating room, as you stare up at the passing ceiling, you are frightened and nervous but confident in the decision that has been made for you.

Now it is 2003, and you have just learned that you have cancer. But this time your doctor does not tell you what to do. Instead, he informs you about the pros and cons of surgery, the pluses and minuses of chemotherapy, and the possibility of treatment with radiation alone. Thank goodness medical science has given us so many options, and thank goodness you have the Internet to boost your knowledge.

But something is wrong. Although you are marvelously well informed, you are having difficulty coming to a decision. The choices are too intricate, the outcomes too uncertain, and your doctor refuses to decide for you. Alone with your Internet reports, you realize you need more than technical information; you need a way to choose between all the complex options, a way to cope with the uncertainty of each, and a way that resonates with your unique personal beliefs and wishes.

CHANGES, CHANGES

Millions of patients have discovered the same unsettling fact: Medical care is no longer simply a matter of following the doctor's instructions. The new complexities of medicine and our changing perceptions of doctors demand our attention and participation in our own medical decisions as never before. And this demand has spawned a plethora of books designed to help the patient-consumer assimilate a growing mountain of medical information.

But as we have seen, there is more to making a medical decision than technical information alone.

The problem is that making medical decisions is not what it used to be. Times have changed, and so have our notions of whom to trust and how to use information. If you are facing a medical decision, you therefore have a crisis on your hands; you are equipped with yesterday's decision tools that function poorly in this new era of medicine.

Medical care and medical decisions have changed.

MEDICAL DECISIONS: NOT WHAT THEY USED TO BE

It used to be easy to make a medical decision. You talked with your doctor, a kindly professional who knew you well for many years, and just followed his or her advice. There were only a few options, and you trusted your doctor to find the right one for you.

But no longer. The rapid progress of medicine has increased the number of our medical options, making them dreadfully complicated. Worse still, even though medical information is more available now than ever before, it is still almost impossible to tell what is real and what is hype. And even if medical data could be quickly and easily understood, our human values—our fears, hopes, and beliefs—are not addressed by sheer information alone. The delivery of medical care is no better; a confusing array of HMOs and insurance companies claim to help expedite our access to medical care, but we can no longer choose our own physicians for ourselves or our children. And because we must face all of this while we are stressed with illness and desperate for information, it is no wonder that each medical decision has become a small crisis.

You will see examples of this crisis wherever you look. There is the college professor searching the Internet night after night to help his father, who is ill with Parkinson's disease. But despite this search, he still does not know what to do, because medical facts alone cannot guide him through the maze of compromises essential to the treatment of this confusing and frustrating disease.

There is the woman with breast cancer who is told to avoid radiation therapy by her trusted doctor of many years. But she is also told she will not live long without it by a famous cancer specialist at a renowned medical school. Whom shall she believe?

There is the middle-aged man with a weak heart and a large family, who must decide between new medications or experimental surgery for his best defense against dropping dead and leaving his young children without a provider.

Surprisingly, the marvelous advancements of medical science have not helped. By giving us so many options, they have made our decisions more complex than ever. And because these options have been created so quickly, there has not been enough time for the thorough testing and comparison required for a rational decision. Modern medicine may have given us many options, but it cannot tell us which to choose.

The most important changes have been those in our attitudes about doctors. We continue to look to them for guidance, but not with the same sense of obedience as before. We have instead empowered ourselves with new responsibilities, arming ourselves with the Internet and a host of new information tools. At times we look to our doctors as we would look to our auto mechanics, expecting them to serve as skilled technicians paid to fix our mechanical bodies without knowing us as human beings. More and more, we find that we are our own medical guides.

The crisis of medical decisions is real. And it is growing, as medical science and societal complexity continue to advance.

Medical decisions are tougher than ever.

Information Is Not Enough

Look through the medical section of your local bookstore and you will find shelf after shelf of books devoted to specific diseases. Books on cancer describe different tumors, graphically depicting the details of surgery and chemotherapy. Books on diabetes exhaustively list the many medications available to keep your blood glucose normal. And books on heart disease tell you how to keep your heart running long and strong.

All these books in their neat rows seem to be telling us something: *Knowledge is power*. They're saying, "Learn all you can about your medical problem, learn all the variations and options, read the right books, and everything will work out. You will conquer the new crisis of medical decisions by acquiring knowledge of your medical problems."

That's great for selling books, but is this really true for making medical decisions? Is the mastery of more and better medical knowledge really all we need to make good medical decisions?

I don't think so. Sure, our decisions are more meaningful when powered with good information than with ignorance. But there is more to a decision than facts. Will a complete and accurate list of diabetes medicines, for example, help us to decide whether we are up to the chore of daily insulin injections? And we must also keep in mind that "facts" can be uncertain, that what is considered true today is often proved false tomorrow.

Most importantly, our decisions must also consider our wishes, needs, expectations, and fears. Simply knowing about a disease and its treatments does not tell you which of these treatments will make you happy. It is a bit like blindly memorizing the road map of the United States; you still need to know where you are, where you want to go, and how much gas it will take to get there.

The same is true for any source of information, whether it be medical books, magazines, or even the powerful Internet. Facts are essential, and this book will devote a good number of pages to showing you how to get them. But meaningful medical decisions require more from us, because facts alone cannot cure the decision crisis. We need other tools, tools that we will develop in the chapters to come.

Knowledge is power. But not enough power.

TWO

The Basic Nature
of Medical Decisions

DISCOVERING you have a medical problem is not a casual event. It is often a turning point that can change your priorities, challenge the way you think, and alter your entire mental world. Making decisions at this time requires a certain patience with these changes and an understanding of their effects upon us. Let's explore this new and sometimes frightening emotional landscape.

YOU ARE NOT ALONE

Having a medical problem is lonely.

Most of us do not consider illness to be a social event. To the contrary, we usually experience illness as an isolation from those around us, withdrawing from others as a cat retires to lick its wounds. And as we withdraw, we begin a journey from the land of the healthy to the land of the sick. The problem is that once we are ill, we are foreigners in both lands, tormented by a loneliness usually reserved for expatriates.

No one feels this more than someone who has just received a serious diagnosis such as cancer. Only moments before, all was normal; but now, with a rude shock, the world has changed to one of surgery and chemotherapy, of fears of pain and humiliation, of thoughts of loved ones after we die. As an inhabitant of the land of the healthy, we cannot sustain such thoughts for long. But as an inhabitant of the land of the sick, we cannot escape them for even a moment. Surrounded by the healthy, who have only to be concerned with the pleasant trivia of making dinner or seeing the latest movies, those with serious illness may feel their isolation swell like an uncontrolled tide.

But objectively speaking, this is all nonsense. Get to know your neighbors, and you will discover innumerable stories of diabetes, or injury, or heart failure, or cancer. We are deceived into thinking we are the only ones with medical problems by our own polite secrecy and by media that insist on depicting only perfect people in perfect health. In a nation hosting more than 70 million surgeries every year, we are surprisingly unaware of even the smallest medical problems of those around us.

Whether the medical decisions you now face are as mundane as the choice of vitamins, or as frightening as choosing treatment for a heart attack, it is natural to feel alone and isolated. But don't allow these feelings to become so distracting that you cannot think about your decisions. Because the fact is, you are not alone. Tough medical decisions are an unavoidable part of life for all of us and are being faced at this very moment by your neighbors, your friends, and the people you see on the street every day. Making medical decisions is a fact of life for everybody.

You are in good company.

YOU ARE NOT YOURSELF

You may have noticed that ever since you learned that you have a medical problem, your mind is not functioning normally. Perhaps you uncharacteristically forgot your doctor's appointment or found yourself daydreaming about medical disasters that may befall you. If your problem is serious enough to threaten your life, you may feel that you are walking around in a daze or you may not be processing information as you normally would. Even issues that are not life threatening such as an impending cosmetic surgery or small alterations in your daily medicine regimen can evoke surprisingly vivid worries. And the fear that often accompanies serious medical problems can virtually paralyze your thoughts and actions.

But remember that these changes are your mind's normal and healthy response to the stress of having a medical problem. Take heart: The dazed feeling will lessen, you will again be more comfortable with information, and you will grow accustomed to minor uncertainties. Depending on your circumstances, the fear you are feeling may not abate, but you will get used to it and you will be able to function despite its uncomfortable and constant presence.

So be patient with yourself through this process. Allow yourself time to accommodate, and forgive yourself for unusual thoughts and behavior. Love yourself, pamper yourself through these difficult times, and you will emerge with the clarity of thought you need to begin making good and sound medical decisions.

Be patient with yourself.

WHAT IS A DECISION?

I was surprised to learn that the word "decide" does not originate from words about the act of choosing. Instead, it comes from a Latin word that means "to cut out." But just what are we cutting when we make our decisions?

Whatever we cut out, we do so hundreds of times each day in hundreds of different ways. We decide when to awaken, which route to take to work, what to eat for dinner. Like these examples, most of our decisions are automatic, straightforward, and of little importance. But decisions are not always this easy. All too often, our decisions are confusing, complex, and at times painful. The decision to take an exciting new job in another city is usually complicated by thoughts of leaving good friends and familiar places. The decision to get married is (one would hope) the result of some serious soul searching. And of course, most medical decisions are charged with the uncertainties and dangers of illness and its treatment.

Decisions do not have to be rational. In fact, most decisions are not based on any obvious serious argument. Why do you brush your teeth before combing your hair? What is it that makes you prefer brunettes to blondes? And as all of us have seen, even important decisions are not always "rational."

So what are we "cutting out" when we make a decision? We are eliminating what we do not choose. If I choose bacon and eggs for breakfast this morning, I lose my bowl of oatmeal. If I vacation in Mexico, I lose my trip to Colorado. And if I choose to treat my tumor with radiation therapy, I lose the comforting finality of surgery.

What defines the significance of our decisions is not what we choose, it is what we have left behind, what we have "cut out" when we make our choices. The ancient roots of the word "decide," therefore, elegantly summarize what is important about our decisions: They demand that something be left behind.

Decisions demand omissions.

WHY DECISIONS HURT

"You can't have your cake and eat it too."

What charges our decisions with emotional conflict is the unhappy reality that hidden within each decision is a loss. In logical terms, if I choose A, I must give up B. A more human example can be found in William Styron's book, *Sophie's Choice*. In this story, a woman and her young daughter and son are caught by the Nazi forces during World War II. Rather than sending both her children to die in the gas ovens, the SS doctor grants Sophie a mind-numbing choice: choose one of her children to die and the other to live. Should she refuse to choose, they will both be sent to die. Stunned and silent, Sophie cannot speak until the doctor begins to lead both children away. She then blurts out, without thinking, "Take my little girl!" Although her choice was granted, the impact of her shattering loss cannot even be imagined.

Although our own decisions may never be this painful, our minds are often tempted to ignore the loss that inevitably and painfully accompanies our medical decisions. For example, if I choose radiation therapy over surgery, I might find myself newly enthusiastic about the benefits of radiation. And I might find that the immediate reaction of my friends and family will be to support my thinking, to confirm the wisdom of my decision. They may avoid any subsequent talk about surgery, and we will distract ourselves with the busy tasks of arranging schedules and appointments. None of us will dwell on what has been lost—the speed, decisiveness, and comforting drama of a surgery. It is usually less frightening to ignore what we have lost when we make a decision than to confront our loss directly.

But the loss nevertheless lingers in our minds. Psychologists tell us that loss creates an undercurrent of anxiety and sadness requiring time to heal, whether we consciously recognize it or not. And they tell us that it is normal to doubt our own decisions, to wonder if we have made the right choice. Decisions are therefore painful for two reasons: the loss of the unchosen option and our nagging doubts about our own wisdom.

There is no way to avoid the losses that are an inevitable part of each of our medical decisions. But the pain can be subdued if we learn to expect loss as a natural consequence of the decision process and if we allow ourselves time enough to recover from those losses we have chosen.

To choose is to lose.

DECISIONS ARE RELATIVE

Not all of our medical decisions are created equal. Some are routine, such as the decision to wear contact lenses or to exercise regularly. Others are more serious, such as whether to treat our cancer with conventional surgery or with an experimental drug. Our decisions may require immediate action, or we may have years for leisurely contemplation. We may be making critical medical decisions for a child or for a parent. Each decision is different, each comes with its own loss, and each has its own nuances of consequences and importance.

Adding to this complexity is the fact that each different type of medical decision may have different meanings for different individuals. A good example of this is the decision facing Stan Q., one of my patients. At age 68, Stan has unfortunately developed lower back pain due to a ruptured disk and a narrowed spinal canal. His pain all but prevents his daily walk to the seniors' center, where he maintains an active social life. Routine chores such as shopping have become more difficult, and his wife cannot help because she herself has been ill at home for many years with congestive heart failure. Medicines have not provided full relief of Stan's pain, and he and I have discussed the possibility of surgery for his condition.

The decision facing Stan is whether to undergo this surgery, which has a good chance of relieving his pain but which also carries a risk (however small) of death or paralysis. After some long and careful thinking, he decided to postpone the surgery. His family, however, did not understand this decision and expressed their frustration to me during a visit to my office. One of his sons said to me, "Why doesn't he just get the operation and get it over with? He wouldn't hurt, and he could do more things for himself and Mom. Sure, there are risks, but there are risks with everything we do. I had a friend who had this surgery and it changed his life."

Although we all sat together in the same small consultation room, Stan did not answer his son directly. Leaning forward slightly, as if to lessen his pain, he instead looked at me squarely and said slowly and deliberately, "I think I'll just live with it for now."

To Stan's son, the operation is simply an unpleasant part of life, a part with guaranteed benefits and only theoretical risks. Perhaps his viewpoint is based on knowledge of the statistics of this operation, or maybe he is a relatively young man with little firsthand experience of life's sadness. Stan, however, is not a young man, and in recent years has lost all too many friends and relatives to illness. He would like some pain relief, but does not want to think what life would be like if he could not leave the house. And there is the issue of his wife, so dependent upon him, who would suffer so much if he became disabled. To Stan's son, the decision for surgery is a no-brainer and will mean improvement; for Stan, this same decision might mean the end of life as he knows it. The facts of the decision are the same for this father and son, but the meaning is completely different. Decisions are relative.

Decisions mean different things to different people. No one else can determine that meaning, and we all know that what is right for one may be wrong for another. At the heart of your decision lies its meaning to you.

You are your own best yardstick.

THREE

Some Philosophical Principles

MAKING A MEDICAL DECISION takes more than a formula. To be sure, we must know something about the Internet and we must be able to contemplate the consequences of our choices. But we must also acknowledge that an effective decision process requires some specific mental attitudes and principles.

REALIZE THAT YOU HAVE DECISIONS

Bob H. is a 45-year-old carpenter who recently learned that he had a problem with his blood pressure. "It's really much higher than it ought to be," said his doctor as he unwrapped the blood pressure cuff from Bob's arm. "You need to be on some medication. Otherwise I'm afraid that you might be headed for a heart attack or a stroke."

"OK, but I really don't feel bad at all," Bob replied, and then smiled. "I'm as healthy as a horse."

"I know, but that's how high blood pressure is," said his doctor, not smiling. "You won't feel a thing until it hits you."

"So what do we do?" asked Bob.

His doctor frowned slightly as he relaxed into his chair behind his desk and reached for a prescription pad. "I'll write you a prescription for this medication. Don't forget to take it twice a day. And I'd like to check your blood pressure again in two weeks."

Many of our medical events seem cut and dried. We have a medical problem; we seek advice from our doctor; we follow instructions. No decisions, no controversy, no hassles. Nice and simple.

But if you look harder, you will discover an almost infinite number of uncertainties and hidden decisions, unavoidable consequences of the complexities of modern medicine. In Bob's case it all seemed very straightforward. But what about the choice of medication? His doctor has selected one, but which of the many available medications will work best? How does his doctor know? Some have side effects such as problems with potassium levels or sexual difficulties. Which of these risks should Bob accept? And should the cost of the medication be a factor in the choice of which to take? Should Bob take more than one medication? Or should he try to treat his high blood pressure with diet and exercise in an attempt to avoid any medication at all? Should he have other tests? Should he consult with other doctors, or with more prestigious medical centers? Is there an operation that he should consider?

I am not trying to sabotage the efforts of your doctors, nor am I suggesting that you spend hours agonizing over every small detail. And I realize how comforting it can be to bring your problems to the doctor and simply follow his or her instructions. But it is important to realize that every medical act requires countless decisions, even if you do not see them all at first glance. How hard you look for them, and what importance you attribute to each, is up to you. But make no mistake: There are always decisions to be made.

There's always a decision to be made.

REALIZE THAT YOU MUST DECIDE

Ritual amputation of the fingers was a medical treatment enthusiastically practiced 25,000 years ago by certain cave dwellers who believed they could magically ward off illness and death by cutting off the fingers of some special but unlucky member of the tribe. The priests in charge of this grisly act must have faced some difficult medical decisions. Which fingers to amputate? When? And how many?

The medical decisions we face in modern times are less gruesome, but there are some similarities. Just as a cave dweller might want to choose for himself which finger to give away, it makes sense that you make your own medical decisions. After all, more is at stake than your fingers.

As obvious as this advice may seem, many people look to others, and especially their doctors, to make all their decisions for them. But even though your doctor is there to help, I think too much of this is a bad idea. True, your doctor is a tremendous source of information and guidance that would be difficult to do without. But no one knows you like you do, no one has your interests at heart as much as you do, and no one else should make each and every one of your decisions. (I will discuss more about our ambivalence about decisions and doctors in chapter eleven.)

There are positive benefits in making your own decisions. Doing so empowers you with a sense of control that can be comforting when you might otherwise feel helpless in the grip of an illness. Accepting the task of deciding will make you more likely to learn the medical facts and more able to achieve the intricate blending of opinions and facts necessary for good decisions. And passivity—waiting to see what happens—can be dangerous. If you don't actively decide, someone else will, and they may be motivated by convenience or cost rather than by what is best for you.

You would not normally entrust another to buy your car, your home, or the clothes you wear without your specific guidance. You shouldn't do that for your medical decisions, either.

Decide for yourself.

REALIZE THAT LIFE IS HARD

"Life ain't made to be easy on folks."
—William Faulkner, *As I Lay Dying*

Well, of course everyone thinks they know this. We all learn that life is coldly unfair and downright hard, and that the perfect life without difficulty is a myth. But in the back of our minds, a voice says, "Except for me." But don't fool yourself; life is indeed hard, for you and me and everybody.

Our modern culture teaches us to believe just the opposite, that life can be perfect if you only know what you are doing. Most of our movies and books have happy endings, in which heroes are rewarded and villains punished. Even the occasional unhappy ending is sweetened with new insights or unanticipated good fortune. Society abhors misfortune.

But some people know and accept life's hard realities. A friend of mine, a physician, had waited for years to retire with his wife so that they could enjoy some family time and travel. I secretly did not want him to retire—he was a good physician, always pleasant, erudite and humorous at the same time. I would miss him. But retire he did, and I was surprised when I saw him walking in the hospital hallways only two weeks later. "What in the world are you doing here?" I teased. "First you dream of going and now you come back. Can't you keep yourself away from work?"

He smiled and pointed to a small, thin woman dressed in hospital pajamas, anchored by plastic tubing to an I.V. pole at the end of the hallway. She was obviously ill, obviously receiving a course of chemotherapy. "My wife," he said. "She just came down with breast cancer, and we are beginning some treatment."

Shocked, I expressed concern, best wishes, and sympathy all at the same time because I knew what hopes he had held for his retirement. Hiding his heartbreak, he only shrugged his shoulders, smiled, and said, "That's life, you know."

As decision makers, we must always be aware that life is hard and unfair. There are no guarantees of good outcomes, no matter how diligent our search for medical facts and insights. We must keep in mind that life can be hard not only for the next guy, but also for us. And when our best efforts end in disaster, we must not blame ourselves. Because, as my friend said, that's life.

Life is hard. Even for you.

Realize That Everything Has Risks

My daily mountain of junk mail always contains plenty of advertisements urging me to take advantage of new "risk-free" investments. I usually throw these away without reading them. For obvious reasons, I hope you do the same.

In medicine as well as the world of finance, there is no such thing as a risk-free strategy. Choosing to ignore your chest pain exposes you to the risk of a further heart attack, choosing surgery has obvious risks, and even the newest of noninvasive treatments for coronary disease have lethal risks of their own.

There are also the hidden risks, the risks of the unexpected. A few people die each year for unknown reasons from the safest of medications. Arteries in the brain can become occluded, unfairly and for no good reason, leading to stroke. As one of my mentors would tell patients when explaining the risks of surgery, "Anything can happen. The chandelier can fall from the ceiling. And I can't predict what will happen to you because I don't have a crystal ball."

The moral: Don't tear your hair out trying to formulate a strategy that is perfectly safe and risk free, because there isn't one. Just having a medical problem means that you have crossed over into a different world and that you will have to accept *some* risk, no matter what you choose to do.

You can't escape risk.

Who Is as Important as *What*

Which would you rather take with you on a hunting trip: A knowledgeable guide who was raised in the area, but no map? Or a complete and detailed map with a guide who couldn't tell north from south?

All but the most stalwart of individualists would rather have a knowledgeable guide than a good map, although having both would be a comfort. Somehow we trust a gifted guide to get us safely to where we need to be, even if done more by intuition than by precision. And we also know that the best of maps is no replacement for true familiarity with the landscape and its inhabitants.

The same is true for medicine. You can gather the most perfect medical data and organize them into the most efficient map of your options and risks, but you won't have the same feel for where to go as does someone who is there every day. And that someone, that gifted guide, is, of course, your doctor.

The problem is that doctors are like guides; some know the territory well, whereas others are well intentioned but seldom visit the places you need to be. And so you need to choose your doctors carefully, not just on the basis of their reputation and demeanor, but on the basis of their demonstrated ability to provide you with guidance, balance, and the wise perspectives born of years of experience.

Finding such a guide is not easy, and no one style fits everyone. Following recommendations of others will help, as will your own intuition. I would also urge you to obtain the help of several doctors, perhaps many if your situation is complex. For just as no one hunting guide can know an entire continent, no doctor can be familiar with every aspect of medicine.

I am not saying to abandon your search for information, nor to stop reading about your medical issues. On the contrary, the more you read and learn, the more likely you are to arrive at a good medical decision. But the ready availability of a mind-boggling mass of medical information means that you need a guide as never before. And whom you choose is of paramount importance, because your choice determines what kind of path you take through the vast wilderness of medical knowledge. Nothing is more powerful than the combination of a good map and a gifted guide.

Find a good guide. And use more than one.

YOU NEED A CAPTAIN OF YOUR SHIP

Lori M. is a 28-year-old woman who discovered she had breast cancer about three years ago and who has made it through the agony of a mastectomy, radiation therapy, and surgery to remove small lumps of cancer in her liver and brain. Despite all of that, she has done well; her baldness is perfectly concealed by her wig and her clothes do not hang as loosely as they have in the past. She remains active and cheerful, and the cancer does not seem to be spreading. I spoke to her recently when she visited my office with her family.

"So how are you?" I asked while observing her speech and movements as she made herself comfortable in her chair.

"I'm doing okay, I guess. Dr. A. said there wasn't much new, and I'm just hanging in there."

Her family smiled and nodded silently at me, pleased with the thought that there was nothing new. Dr. A. was Lori's primary physician, a very competent and caring doctor with whom I had worked many times before.

"Are you scheduled for a follow-up MRI? And are you still taking steroids?" I asked. I wanted to make sure we didn't overlook any new tumors, and I wanted to be sure she didn't take steroids for too long because of potentially serious side effects.

"Well, Dr. X. said the MRI was up to you. I don't know about the steroids; Dr. Y. gave them to me and I haven't seen him since the last surgery."

I wasn't too happy when I heard this. She should have had her MRI two months ago, and that delay could give a new cancer the opportunity to grow unchecked. It also appeared that even though so many doctors were involved in her last surgery, no one had taken the primary responsibility of fine-tuning her steroids.

Despite the help of many good doctors and a concerned family, Lori had fallen into the cracks of the medical system. Her medical problems were so complex that her medical care had become fragmented among specialists, and no one person had been appointed to guide her through the pieces. She found herself bouncing from one doctor to another, each of them assuming that one of the others had a watchful eye on the big picture. She was adrift in a medical ocean, drifting on a ship with no captain.

Lori's problem can happen to anyone, anywhere, even in the best of medical centers. Complex medical problems with many options are common, and it is easy to get lost in a web of specialists. Nor does simply having a family doctor help, since he or she may feel a need to fade into the background as the specialists take over.

And here's the surprising part: This is a problem that your doctors cannot be trusted to solve, for they are themselves part of the problem.

The solution must come from you, and to solve it I suggest you take three steps.

1. Realize that you need a captain of your medical ship, and then choose one. This could be your family doctor or one of your specialists, such as an oncologist or cardiologist.
2. Talk with this doctor and say frankly that you need a primary doctor to organize your total medical care, to have your big picture always in view. Don't be timid. Your doctor will welcome this opportunity and will be flattered by your trust.
3. Take the responsibility to visit and contact this doctor frequently, so that your medical circumstances can be reviewed often and modified as needed. No one can be a good captain without a ship.

Asking for a captain is an important and reasonable request, necessary to your health. Don't go to sea without one.

Find a captain.

DON'T FIGHT YOURSELF

We have said before that illness is a frightening and disorienting experience, altering our behavior and muddling our thoughts. But no matter what happens to you, you are at heart the same person. No matter how strange and unfamiliar your medical problems may be, you are the same person as before, with the same attitudes, emotions, and style. If you have always been naturally cautious and suspicious of dramatic risks, you may choose to defer surgery to remove your deep-seated tumor. Your natural instincts will be more comfortable waiting until the CT scan or the MRI shows that the tumor is growing before electing surgical treatment. On the other hand, if taking thought-out risks has always given you a sense of comfort and control, you may be more comfortable having the surgery to remove this "time bomb" within you. How you are put together determines which decisions are comfortable, and how you are does not change just because you have a medical problem.

We do not magically change our personalities and preferences when we become ill; rather, we are the same old people with new problems.

Remember that, and do not expect yourself to change to fit someone else's notion of style. Be true to the feelings and motivations that you have always had in the past.

Don't push square pegs into round holes.

TAKE SOME BREAKS

Football games have half times, basketball games have quarters. Even professional athletes need breaks in the most heated of events.

And you are no exception. No human being can sustain the mental tension of coping with tough medical decisions twenty-four hours a day, seven days a week. To remain healthy and focused, you must take some breaks and find periodic relief from your emotional burden.

Writers know this, as do mathematicians and artists. They know that some of their most profound insights occur during moments of relaxation, when their thoughts are far from their professional tasks. While it is crucial to concentrate on what you are doing and the goals you want, periodic breaks renew the mind and spirit and pave the way for inspiration. It is as if the mind requires release to seek its own solutions.

A total break from the anxiety and worry of a medical problem is often not possible. But go through the motions anyway. The anxiety may not lift completely, but the act of doing something different and enjoyable will be refreshing.

You may feel guilty if you take a break, or be frightened that you will miss something important if you allow your mind to wander from your problems, even for a minute. But you must admit that a few minutes or even hours every day will not matter if you are otherwise focused. You have the time.

Your breaks should be fun. Do whatever it is that you like to do, anything to escape for a short while. Watch movies, make dinner, visit friends, travel. You can even pretend briefly that you are carefree. A glass of wine may help. But do something.

Breaks are important. They rejuvenate the soul and they make life worth living during your struggle with your medical problems.

Be kind to yourself. Take a break.

Part II
The Six Steps of
Medical Decision Making

FOUR

An Introduction to the Six Steps of Medical Decision Making

WHEN PRESENTED with a troubling medical diagnosis, it may seem at first that we are being bombarded all at once with issues and questions at all levels:

Where can I find medical information?

How does it relate to my situation?

Which parts of it should I believe?

How do I assess risk, staying calm and focused?

What is the place for statistics?

What sort of help do I need, and from whom?

How do we make sense of this chaos? Over the years I have observed and helped and struggled along with my patients to find a way through this confusion, to find paths to decisions that make sense both medically and personally. Based on these observations, I have organized the decision process into six steps. Not everyone will take each step, and not everyone will take each step in order. But these six steps are so fundamental to good decision making that I am convinced they will be helpful—even crucial—to you.

Much has been written about how people make decisions, because decision making plays such a critical role in the fundamental activities of economics, politics, and business. No one theory explains every decision, of course, since many types of decisions are made under an infinite variety of circumstances. Some are made spontaneously and quickly, defying all logic; others are made only after months of deliberate mathematical calculations. In this section we will take a few lessons from the theory of decisions, and in the next section we will see how these lessons lead to our six-step plan.

How We Decide: The Theory

Philosophers tell us that decisions are motivated by three forces: our desires, our beliefs, and the meaning that the decision has for us. Let's look at each of these forces as they relate to our medical decision making.

The desire behind a decision is simply the motivation leading us (or forcing us) to decide. For example, a patient with diabetes might be motivated to decide between pills and insulin if he wants to avoid the complications of this disease.

Our beliefs are the second important force behind our decision process, because a decision is always based on beliefs about its consequences. Continuing the above example, I may believe that daily insulin injections are absolutely necessary to maintain my blood sugar levels, and I may believe that my health will suffer if my blood sugar is too high. I may also have certain beliefs about the complications of insulin or of pills. Beliefs do not have to be based on cold, hard facts in order to be useful. Those rooted in faith and subjectivity are as important and as essential to our decisions as those based on facts.

The inclusion of subjective meaning into our decision process is the final crucial ingredient. For example, the decision whether to take insulin or adopt a rigorous diet-and-exercise schedule might be tempered by the personal meaning attached to daily insulin injections. For some, injections are seen as just another minor inconvenience, far less intrusive than a massive change in lifestyle. For others, injections are a symbol of dependence on drugs and can evoke unpleasant childhood memories of shots and doctors. Even drastic changes in diet and exercise would seem better than this daily ordeal.

In just this simple scenario, differences in subjective meaning lead to different medical decisions, even without consideration of efficacy or risk. Meaning is powerful indeed.

Decisions are made of motives, information, beliefs, and meanings.

HOW WE DECIDE: A PRACTICAL SIX-STEP PLAN

"Life is a long trip in a cheap car. In a dark country. Without a good map."
—Frederic Schick, *Making Choices*

If life is a long, dark road, then the path to good medical decisions may be one of its more tortuous routes. But as for any trip, a little planning goes a long way. Building on our view of decisions as composed of information, beliefs, and meanings, we can see the elements we need to arrive at our decisions. We need to know which roads are open (our options) and where they lead (the tradeoffs inherent in their pros and cons). We need to gather data about each road and know how to interpret what we find. We also need to take stock of our beliefs about what each road might hold for us and to think about the personal meaning of each imagined destination.

And so we have listed our six steps of medical decision making: identification of options; identification of tradeoffs; discovery of data; interpretation of data; gathering of beliefs; and contemplation of meaning. We will take a brief look at each of these steps here, then address each step in detail later on.

STEP 1: IDENTIFICATION OF YOUR OPTIONS

It seems simple enough; before you can make your medical decisions, you must know what your choices are. But discovery of every possible choice often takes work and ingenuity. I believe that this work is so important that it deserves to be our first step in making medical decisions.

You will probably discover that many possibilities are open to you, including several types of surgery, chemotherapy, medications, or other treatments. Your possibilities may also include experimental therapies at specialized centers. And don't forget that choosing no treatment is always an option.

Do not be judgmental at first in your search for options. Your task at this point is to ferret out all the possibilities, not to judge them. Save critical evaluation for later. Go ahead and make note of the weird therapy using eggshell extracts and the experimental radiation that sounds so dangerous. You can scratch them off the list later. For now, let them all pour in.

Where can you find a complete list of your options? Not in any one place. Your doctor is a good place to start because he or she will review many of your options with you. But don't stop there. As elsewhere in this book, I urge you to consult with several doctors, adding specialists depending on the complexity of your problem. You may hear options from one doctor that you do not from another.

But don't stop there, either. Reading about your medical problems and digging through medical articles, books, and the Internet is a great strategy to find other options, and I will show you later how to use these resources effectively and quickly. Other options may arise from discussions with your friends or from the newspaper and television. Use all your resources.

The first important step in making a medical decision is to know what is possible. We will address this crucial task in detail in chapter five.

Know your possibilities.

STEP 2: IDENTIFICATION OF TRADEOFFS

There is no such thing as a perfect solution. Or a perfect medical option.

Once you have identified all your medical options, the next step is to compare them with one another with the hope of choosing the best one. What you will learn quickly is that no option is perfect and that each has some rather serious pros and cons. You will therefore have to make some compromises and tradeoffs.

Consider, for example, the choice between surgery or radiation treatment for prostate cancer. More is involved here than a simple consideration of which treatment works best. In some cases, surgery may have the advantage of a longer survival time, but it may also have the drawback of a greater risk of sexual impotence. The choice is really a decision about tradeoffs: survival *versus* quality of life.

Other examples abound. Heart surgery may prolong life, but may also require restriction of physical activity in the future. Use of anticoagulants ("blood thinners" to slow formation of blood clots) reduces the risk of lethal pulmonary emboli but increases the risk of fatal bleeding into the brain after even a minor fall. Hysterectomy may be needed to treat certain benign tumors, but then, of course, childbearing is impossible.

After identifying your options, the next step is to identify the pros and cons of each. Again, this will require some reading and discussions with your doctors. And as before, this is not the time to be judgmental or eliminate certain options before further consideration. List all the pros and cons and you will be ready to choose between them in later steps. We'll cover this step in detail in chapter six.

Find the compromises.

STEP 3: DISCOVERY OF DATA

Seeing the difficult tradeoffs is only the beginning. You must then get down to the hard task of evaluating each of the options and tradeoffs that you so laboriously found. But how?

There are many ways to assess your options, but what you need first are hard facts. Opinions are certainly useful, especially from your doctors, but that will come later. Right now we are only interested in data.

Unlike other fields, there are few absolutes in medicine. No one can predict that a particular treatment will always succeed, and no one can promise that complications will never occur. Medical facts are therefore usually expressed as a percentage; a 75% chance of survival after surgery for breast cancer, or a 12% risk of sudden death from a particular heart medication. Our search for real data is therefore really a search for percentages. And the discovery of these percentages constitutes our third step of medical decision making.

Finding medical data is difficult. It requires a resolute attitude, a consistent strategy, and a certain expertise in navigating medical writing. I will show you how in chapter seven.

Good data are worth the effort.

STEP 4: INTERPRETATION OF NUMBERS

Do you remember what it was like the last time you bought a car? You probably looked at car prices in the newspaper ads, or looked in special books of car prices or on the Internet. Then you went to the car dealership and listened to the salesman tell you the price of the car you wanted.

Did you believe everything you heard?

Of course not. You knew that the prices you found in ads or from salesmen might not be the real price needed to buy the car. And you knew that data obtained from salesmen are best received with a certain amount of interpretation.

I wish that medicine were different. I wish that finding medical data was all we needed to make good medical decisions And I wish that all we had to do was simply to pick the option with the greatest chance of success and lowest risk of problems.

But we must do more.

The problem is that medical data cannot be accepted at face value. While one scientific study might conclude that the risk of surgical complications for an operation is 80%, another might demonstrate only a 10% risk of the same complication. And the reasons for this difference might be difficult to see; there may have been subtle errors in one of the studies, or the type of patients might be different in each study, or there may have been small but important differences in how the operation was performed at each hospital. There are thousands of possible sources of error and differences in medical data.

We must not only find medical facts, we must also interpret them. We must evaluate their sources and decide which facts we can safely believe. This is not always easy, because medical facts are frequently incomplete and contradictory. Scientists spend major portions of their careers agonizing over which facts to believe and which to discard. But we must do this in the limited time we have for our own medical decisions.

And so this important task is both complex and difficult. In chapter eight, I will show you in detail how to begin the interpretation of your medical data. We cannot, of course, include a complete mathematical course on statistics. But I will show you some tricks and ways of thinking that will help you decide for yourself what is believable and what is not.

Be skeptical.

STEP 5: GATHERING YOUR BELIEFS

Unfortunately, facts and numbers are not enough to guide us to the right medical decision. To be sure, facts and numbers are essential, and acquiring them is worth our best efforts. But many questions remain that defy resolution with facts alone. How long will I live (not statistically, but really)? Are alternative therapies better than standard medicine? What kind of vitamins should I be taking, if any? How far can I trust the medical delivery system? How far should I trust my doctor?

These important questions can only be answered when we take stock of our beliefs. We might, for example, believe in our hearts that there is something inherently harmful about radiation therapy. There is certainly evidence for this view. But there is also strong evidence against it, and neither viewpoint is completely true. Our beliefs therefore serve us not so much as statements of immutable fact but more as guiding beacons through an otherwise dark sea of contradictory facts. Our beliefs about the proper role of physicians, about the strength of mind-body connections, and about family and religion are also clearly central in how we go about finding medical decisions.

Beliefs are powerful. Imagine the effect upon your life and your decisions if you truly believed that you would die when you finished reading this paragraph. Beliefs can also be wrong, as when most people believed the world to be flat. But most of the beliefs we hold about medical issues cannot be said to be right or wrong; they are instead valuable assessments of complex issues that we have been forced to make when the facts are unavailable, contradictory, or irrelevant.

I am not saying that you should stick to your beliefs no matter what, or that you should never critically examine why you believe what you do. In fact, it would be unhealthy (if not pigheaded) if we did not occasionally examine our beliefs, changing them as facts became more clear, or at least softening them to fit new data. After all, very few still believe that the world is flat. But all too often, the facts cannot fully address the important questions, and it is then that your beliefs become your most valuable barometer.

Let's look at an example that may make this clear. Nancy is a 68-year-old woman in remarkably good health, who began experiencing excruciating facial pain that she described as "like someone taking a hot poker and jabbing it into my cheek." The name for her problem is trigeminal neuralgia, a condition most likely caused by pulsations of an artery in the brain that irritate the sensory nerve to the face. This condition is not life threatening, but is so painful that it has been known to provoke suicide. As happens to many with her ailment, Nancy's medicines were no longer working and she came to my office to discuss surgery.

There are three types of surgery for trigeminal neuralgia. The first is a major surgery called a microvascular decompression, in which the back of the skull is opened to gently reposition the offending artery away from the nerve. In most cases, this eliminates the pain and has no side effects. The second type of operation does not deal with the artery directly. Instead, a needle is inserted through the cheek and threaded through a hole at the base of the skull to deaden the nerve with electricity, chemicals, or mechanical pressure. This operation is also effective at relieving the pain, but results in a numbness of the face that can be uncomfortable. The third type of surgery is radiosurgery, in which a beam of radiation is used to damage the nerve. Although this method requires no needles and no incisions, it doesn't work as often as the other operations and requires the use of radiation.

I explained these alternatives to Nancy, presenting them all as reasonable options with different pros and cons. On the face of it, then, Nancy had a choice among three relatively evenly matched operations.

The microvascular decompression offered the best chance of pain relief without side effects but was a major operation; the needle procedure worked well but resulted in a numb face; and radiosurgery was less invasive but involved radiation. Nancy's health was excellent, so microvascular decompression seemed to be her best choice.

But Nancy had other beliefs that were as important to her as my factual comparison of these three operations. Despite her health, she believed that her age and general condition would make her more prone to serious complications from a big operation like microvascular decompression. And despite the statistical safety of this procedure, the medical facts did not allow me to assure her with complete certainty that nothing bad would happen. Both Nancy and I knew medical statistics were just that; statistics that could not foretell the future for any one particular patient.

For unclear reasons, Nancy also believed that treatment with radiation would lead to bad results, perhaps cancer or nerve damage, although she could not be exactly sure. Again, I told her about the scientific studies that have been done and about the low risk of complications with radiation. But something inside her told her that radiation was likely bad, and that something was her belief that radiation would do more harm than good.

So what did Nancy do? She chose to undergo the percutaneous needle procedure and to accept the inevitable facial numbness that would result. I think that in some "objective" sense, the microvascular decompression would have been better for her, because it offered the same pain relief without facial numbness and at a very low risk. Likewise, I do not share her beliefs that radiation treatments will always lead to harm. But I have to admit that no facts or figures can absolutely prove her wrong, although they might sway a different person with different beliefs. I may not agree with Nancy's beliefs about the risks of surgery or the nature of radiation, but her decision was based on beliefs that she held at a very fundamental level. For that reason, I think she made the right choice.

Incidentally, Nancy did undergo the percutaneous procedure and did very well. Her pain is gone, and she only rarely notices her facial numbness.

Beliefs are painfully individual, painful because we all have had the embarrassing experience of our most cherished beliefs being ridiculed by others. But we must nevertheless be honest with ourselves about what it is we believe. For our beliefs are an important part of who we are, of what we have experienced and learned in our lifetimes, and enable us to confront difficult situations with limited facts. To be sure, we must be flexible enough to change our beliefs when the evidence seems compelling, and we will consider this process in detail in chapter nine. But our beliefs are a part of us and should not be ignored in our medical decisions.

Pay attention to your beliefs.

STEP 6: CONTEMPLATION OF MEANING

This is the final step of our plan for good medical decision making. Let's suppose we have identified our tradeoffs, found and interpreted some data that describe their efficacy and safety, and examined our beliefs about the nature of the tradeoffs and their implications. Now we have to make the actual choice between surgery or radiation, or between insulin or pills, and it may seem like there is still something missing. That something is a consideration of the subjective meaning of the decision.

What is the meaning of a decision? It is the subjective value that the decision has for you, a personal assessment of the emotional and practical consequences of this decision on your life. The same decision will have different meanings for different people, depending on their circumstances and personalities.

An example may make this clear. Howard K. is a 52-year-old retired insurance executive who developed a bad tremor in his arms and hands about four years ago that seems to be slowly worsening. He has what is called an essential tremor, a tremor that is often severe but rarely life threatening. As is not uncommon, medicines did not work, so Howard had come to talk with me about surgical ways to control his tremor.

It turns out that there is a relatively new operation that improves this particular tremor about 70% of the time, called deep brain stimulation, or DBS. In this procedure, a wire is inserted very precisely into a small area deep within the brain and connected under the skin to a pacemaker. The pacemaker is kept on for most of the day, stimulating the part of the brain at the tip of the wire. Almost miraculously, most of the time the tremors will vanish or dramatically diminish as soon as the stimulator is turned on.

I told all of this to Howard and his family and described the technical details of the operation, which involves computers, CT scans, and head frames. We discussed the 1 or 2 % risk of death or catastrophe and the risks of arm weakness and difficulties with walking. I warned him of the need to return periodically for programming of the stimulator, and of the need for another operation every few years to replace the stimulator battery. He seemed to understand all of this and accepted it calmly.

But the real crux of the conversation came when I asked him to describe to me what effects the tremor had upon him. As he spoke, his voice became hoarse and his eyes filled with tears. His tremor, which caused his arms to fling wildly and unpredictably, prevented him from dressing himself, or feeding himself without destroying the kitchen. Howard had been the strong backbone of his family, so that his needs for help in dressing and grooming, or requiring a straw to eat dinner were humiliating and demoralizing. But there was more. Howard had been an avid woodcarver for years and had looked forward to really enjoying this hobby after he retired. But the tremor had ruined these plans, and his workshop remained idle. Finally, Howard's difficulties at meals were so embarrassing at restaurants and parties that he and his wife found themselves now in almost complete social isolation. It was no wonder, then, that Howard chose to undergo DBS implantation.

On the other hand, Peter K. is a 65-year-old farmer who has the same type of tremor as Howard, with the same severity and quality. Peter is still active around the family farm, although his sons handle the brunt of the chores and business arrangements. Peter's duties are rather physical, so that he does not find that the tremor gets in his way. He does not seem to mind being careful at dinner and using a straw, nor is his social life affected, because most of his time is spent on the farm with his family. He came to my office only through the persistent urging of his neurologist, eyeing me suspiciously as I recited the details of the operation and its risks, as I had for Howard. At the end, he looked slowly at his family, turned to me, and pronounced, "I guess I'll just think about it for a bit." Both Peter and I knew that he wanted no part of that operation. As he left my office, I smiled, for I believed that he had made the right choice.

The difference between these two men is not the nature of their tremor, nor their assessment of the efficacy and risks of the operation, nor their belief system. The difference is the meaning that the tremor and its treatment has for each of them. For Howard, the tremor means a disruption of his social life, his retirement hopes, and his standing in his family. Accepting the risks, uncertainties, and inconveniences of treatment, therefore, makes a lot of sense. For Peter, however, the tremor is just another nuisance of aging and has little impact on his activities or social life. I would have been surprised (and resistant) had he chosen the surgery.

The meaning that a medical decision has for us cannot be calculated from a formula or measured with a medical test. Nor can meaning be found in books, because the meaning of a disease or its treatment depends on our own special circumstances and temperament. There is no one right answer, no one right decision that can be found by consulting a computer algorithm; the quality that makes a decision right is the meaning it has for us. This is why I have called this sixth component of our plan the contemplation of meaning; we must reflect within ourselves to find meaning that is real for us. Only in this last and most important step can we see to make individual medical decisions that make sense.

Decisions are meaningless without meaning.

FIVE

Step 1: Identification of Your Options

WE BEGIN the process of making a medical decision by finding all available options. We will evaluate them later; the task at hand is just to list each and every medical possibility available to you. As we will see, this requires some work.

USE YOUR SOURCES

You may not realize it, but you already have access to a surprising number of sources of medical information. Your doctor, of course, is an important source, and so are any specialists involved in your care. But don't forget that your friends and family are also valuable sources, especially if they're on the lookout for helpful information. Newspapers, radio, and television constantly cover medical items of interest and can be strong sources. Even television dramas can clue you in to medical alternatives you might otherwise miss.

We will show you how to use these sources in great detail once we get to chapter seven. For now, I urge you to begin using these sources to find your options, leaving criticism of each option for later. You will be surprised at the number of ideas and possibilities that you can discover as you talk with your friends, watch television, search the Internet, and read medical articles. Take these ideas to your doctors, read and search some more, and talk with your doctors again. Keep at it, use all your sources, and you may find important options that were not evident at first glance.

Use all your tools.

CAN I REALLY TALK TO MY DOCTORS?

Let's face it, visiting the doctor is intimidating for anyone. After all, you don't know as much as the doctor, and you wouldn't be there if he or she didn't have more medical power than you do.

But don't fall into the trap of letting these normal feelings of intimidation prevent you from having a straightforward talk with your doctor. Some people become so passive and frightened that they will not ask questions and so cannot obtain explanations from their physician, and they would rather sink into the ground than challenge the doctor's advice. And some doctors encourage this unfortunate distance, because they are too busy or too distracted or just plain mean.

Should you talk with your doctor? Yes. Should you overcome your awkwardness and fears and ask your questions? Yes. Should you challenge his or her advice if it seems not to make sense? Yes. Should you expect clear explanations and meaningful discussions? Yes, yes, yes.

Remember, this is *your* show. This is all about you—your health, your problems, even your life. Your doctor is not your friend, and his or her feelings are immaterial. You are there to get well, not to go with the flow. So if you find you cannot talk meaningfully with your doctor despite your best efforts, don't hesitate to find another.

Talk with your doctor.

KEEP AN OPEN MIND

You are talking to your cousin Ralph about your problems with high blood pressure, and he insists on telling you about a new banana extract that is supposed to be good for controlling this pernicious problem.

Or you happen to watch a soap opera and see a new type of renal dialysis machine that seems to be better than the one used for you. Or you read in the newspaper that a new form of meditation is being tried for the treatment of chronic pain.

You will come across all sorts of ideas as you search for your medical options. Some are truly silly, but others only seem bizarre until you investigate further. And it is often impossible to tell at first glance what is ridiculous and what might be lifesaving. What I suggest, therefore, is that you postpone judgment of what you find until later in your search for a decision. Take note of all ideas, even the ones that seem farfetched. You can eliminate the bad ideas later, after you have looked into them in more detail.

And you never know. That banana extract just might work.

Listen now, check it out later.

WHERE TO GO FOR YOUR MEDICAL CARE

Rebecca W. is a 38-year-old university professor who learned that she had ovarian cancer. After the initial shock of this devastating news had lessened, she spoke with her doctors and searched the Internet to learn which types of surgery and chemotherapy would be best for the treatment of her disease. It seemed fairly standard, and all the main options were available at the university center where she worked. She decided to stay there for her medical treatment.

To her horror and frustration, her tumor continued to grow despite surgery and chemotherapy. More desperate now, she continued to search and found other alternatives. The first was a naturopathic cancer center located in the mountains above the city where Rebecca lived. This center used natural diet, exercise, meditation, and imagery to combat cancer. The second was a medical center specializing in cancer located in a major city 1,500 miles away. This center had an aggressive approach to surgery and was renowned for the novel ways it used chemotherapy to treat ovarian cancer. The third alternative was a medical center in Europe that sponsored several experimental trials for the treatment of her type of ovarian cancer.

Rebecca discovered an interesting but rarely appreciated fact about modern medicine: Things are not the same everywhere. To be sure, some aspects of medical care are standardized and accepted throughout the world. No one would amputate your hand to treat a heart attack, for example. But medicine is closer to an art than a science, so that the basic tools of surgery and medications are used differently in different places. And this can matter a great deal.

This means that one of the most important categories you should include on your list of options is the location of your medical care. Your list might include care at your neighborhood hospital, or at one of several major centers in your city, or at specialized centers around the country or around the world, or at centers for alternative medicine. Your choice is much more than a choice of location; it is a selection of a particular set of resources, expertise, and philosophy in the treatment of your medical problem. Needless to say, think about them all and choose carefully.

In my opinion, even if you are determined to obtain your care in your own neighborhood, you should investigate other centers. If nothing else, you might learn about other new and important options that might otherwise have escaped you. These new treatments might be carried out near home, although you may ultimately decide to go elsewhere. I also suggest that you discuss the pros and cons of other centers with your doctors. A good doctor will not be threatened by your interest, and you may learn some striking advantages (or disadvantages) of these other centers.

One advantage of receiving care in your own city is, of course, the convenience of avoiding travel. You'll also have your family and other support close by. Using a local medical center can also be a big advantage if you require daily treatment or frequent return visits. On the other hand, a large medical center in a distant city may have expertise and experience with your medical problems that may make a difference. In that case, the trouble and expense of travel, missed work, and hotel bills may be worth the effort. These problems may be easier if you have friends or relatives in this distant city, and you can sometimes arrange to receive specialized care at a distant center combined with routine care in your own city.

I realize that the practicalities of travel may prevent you from receiving care elsewhere. Most of us find travel to be difficult, and many cannot afford the great expense of a prolonged trip even if it has life-saving potential. This is not right or fair, but is often a sad reality. One option is to sell the farm—to desperately marshal all possible resources no matter what the cost. But this is rarely necessary, and you should not choose such a sacrifice without a great deal of thought and advice from family, friends, and doctors. Another alternative is to ask your doctors to consult with the other medical center, to obtain some other opinions and ideas. It is not unheard of, for example, for a new chemotherapy regimen to be given at a local hospital with the help of advice from a medical center far away. You can still benefit from outside medical expertise even if you are unable to travel.

One caveat: Just because a medical center is famous does not mean it is the center for you, and you may need to explore several major institutions before finding just the right one. Lance Armstrong, for example, in his inspiring book, *It's Not About the Bike*, tells the story of his search for medical care after learning he had developed testicular cancer. He was quickly referred to a major hospital specializing in cancer, but the doctors there seemed dispassionate, and the treatment they proposed did not take into account his desire to continue as a world-class cyclist. After some digging around and after much soul searching with his friends and family, he decided to transfer his care to another major center that offered not only a deep experience with his type of cancer but also a sensitivity to his wishes for his future. The rest—his winning the Tour de France, not once, but *five times*, after his cancer —is history.

The choice of where you receive your care is crucial, because location can either open new options or limit your possibilities. Make this choice with care, using all your sources of information. And don't be afraid to change locations if that seems like the right thing to do.

Location, location, location.

HOW TO FIND AND BE SEEN AT OUTSIDE MEDICAL CENTERS

It doesn't take a crystal ball to locate medical centers specializing in your problem, and it doesn't take a magic key to get in. All you need is a little time spent asking around, some Internet work, and a few phone calls.

Ask your doctor. He or she will know the good places, or know someone who does. And your doctor can make arrangements (the *referral*) for you to be seen at other centers. Don't be shy; most doctors understand your concerns and want to help. And if your doctor seems miffed or insulted, it's time to find another doctor. After all, this is about your health, not your doctor's feelings.

Ask around. Your friends and family will have abundant opinions about where to go and whom to see. Not all of these opinions are well founded, of course, but they can make you aware of medical centers that you might not find otherwise.

Ask the Internet. I will show you how to find reliable Web sites that address your medical problems in chapter seven, and most of these Web sites contain links to medical centers offering specialized expertise.

Call the medical centers that seem best. Don't think for a minute that you are not worthy to call the Greatest Medical Center on Earth. To the contrary, you are indispensable to these centers, you are what they exist for—they need you and they need your business. Don't be afraid to make contact. They are waiting for you.

A final small bit of extra advice, a lagniappe. When you make contact with the other center, when you are talking with a real person on the phone, ask for other ideas or places. Sure, they work for the hospital, but they are familiar with the terrain and most often they will be nice enough to tell you what they know.

Seek and ye shall find.

The Small-Town Syndrome

There is a corollary to the advice of the last section. Don't stay at home if the medical care is better somewhere else.

I have seen this many times. A patient living in a small town will choose to stay in that town for medical treatment, no matter how complex the medical issues. It is more convenient to obtain local care, friends and family are nearby, and the local doctors are well known and trusted.

But even though many small towns contain superb medical facilities, it has always made sense to me to seek an opinion for complex medical problems at one of the many major medical centers located across the country. And as a rule of thumb, the more serious your diagnosis, the more you should consider outside expertise. Even if you go only for a second opinion, it is often well worth the time and money. Medicine is a complex and changing art form, so that what was intractable yesterday might be curable today. And don't hesitate to contact the big-name centers; they will welcome your call because they exist to help patients like yourself.

It's your health; you owe it to yourself to take the best of what medicine has to offer.

Don't be afraid to travel.

Whom to Choose for Your Medical Care

Much has been written about how to choose a doctor or other medical practitioner, so I will only touch on a few points here. Whom you choose to provide your medical care will obviously determine many of your options. A naturopathic healer will suggest a different course of treatment for your foot pain than a podiatrist, and an orthopedic surgeon may suggest even more options than a podiatrist. Which general type of practitioner you choose will be based on your beliefs and opinions, but don't forget to use your information sources to identify a nice variety of choices.

I would suggest that you choose your doctor with at least as much care as you choose your car mechanic.

Consider the doctor's reputation. The best way to do this is to ask other doctors and any friends (or friends of friends) you may have in the medical profession. Local word of mouth reputation is usually (but not always!) accurate. You can also ask other patients, but be aware that even the worst doctors have a faithful following.

Visit with the doctor and trust your instincts. Are you comfortable that you are being heard and your problems being helped? Does your doctor seem to be competent and compassionate? No one style fits everyone, and your gut feelings are valuable in this assessment.

Don't be afraid to use more than one doctor, especially if you have complex medical problems. One doctor should be in charge of your general care, but specialists can expand the options available to you.

And as I have said before, don't worry about hurting your doctor's feelings when you ask for other opinions.

Your doctor is often a gatekeeper to medical options. Choose wisely.

Be smart about whom you choose.

BE ON THE LOOKOUT

Like any opportunity, a medical option may arise unexpectedly. You may hear of a new medication effective against kidney stones just as you decide for surgery, or you may discover an experimental trial for diabetes after you have been taking insulin for years. Medicine is a moving target, changing from year to year as new advances surface. Be on the lookout for new options; you're bound to find some.

Keep your eyes peeled for options.

SIX

Step 2: Identification of Tradeoffs

NOW THAT YOU HAVE IDENTIFIED your medical options, the second step of our plan is to compare them all in the hope of finding the best one. At times, the pros and cons of each option are obvious. But sometimes a different type of thinking is needed to really see the important advantages and disadvantages. This chapter will show you some tips and techniques to make that possible.

YOU'VE BEEN FRAMED!

Would you like to win the lottery?

Sure you would. More money, security, and luxury for life. Who wouldn't want to win? But humor me for just a moment, and try to think of all the reasons you would *not* want to win all that sumptuous money. Sounds crazy, but here goes.

All that money would be difficult to manage, and there would be tremendous pressure not to lose it. It would be hard to make new friends who like you for yourself and not your wealth. Old friends might suddenly appear and expect financial support. And it might be more difficult to be truly happy.

What makes this exercise interesting, if not uncomfortable, is that we deliberately tried to unseat some of our assumptions about money. These assumptions are part of our normal mental framework that we habitually use when thinking about finances, and may seem obvious. The assumption that more money is a good thing is rarely challenged. Our exercise was an attempt to think outside of this framework.

Social psychologists call this collection of assumptions a "frame." Just as we look outside of our homes through the frame surrounding our windows, so do we view different aspects of reality with different mental frames. And the view through different frames can be surprising. Our normal thoughts about money, for example, were once challenged in a study conducted by some social scientists who wondered if lottery winners were always happy. They made the surprising discovery that lottery winners were no happier than paralyzed victims of traffic accidents after one year. Their frame shift allowed them to anticipate an otherwise completely unexpected result.

A famous example of how frames can affect our thinking is the common metaphor of the half-empty glass. A pessimist sees the glass as half empty; an optimist sees it as half full. The facts are the same, but our interpretation depends on how we frame them.

Let's look at an example of how frames can affect our medical decisions. Arteriovenous malformations (AVMs) are abnormalities in the brain consisting of tangles of blood vessels that look like masses of spaghetti buried within the brain tissue. Normally silent, an AVM is dangerous because it can bleed suddenly and unexpectedly, producing a major stroke or even death. Fortunately, the risk of such a bleed is small, only about 3 to 4% per year.

How this risk is told to a patient can irrevocably frame the issue forever. If the physician says, "You've got a time bomb in your head. The risk of it exploding is small, but no one knows when or if it will go off," you can bet that surgery will be chosen, and fast. If, on the other hand, the physician smiles and says, "Great news! There is no need for surgery. The risk of bleeding is not zero, and I can't guarantee that it won't happen, but the risk is very small," surgery will probably be postponed. The danger is now framed as an escape from a risky surgery instead of as a bomb. Same facts, different frames, but a vastly different picture.

Here's another example. Mark W. is a 42-year-old high school coach who went to his doctor for headaches that were waking him at night. To his horror, an MRI scan showed a small tumor in his brain next to his skull.

Mark is an aggressive and competitive sportsman, so it was no surprise that he launched an all-out attack on the medical literature to find the best treatment for his tumor. He learned that surgery and chemotherapy are the best tools, and he talked at length with his doctor about which option to choose. He wanted action. After much discussion and many sleepless nights, Mark and his wife finally decided that Mark would have surgery, and they visited a neurosurgeon.

Mark was shocked to hear the surgeon suggest he have no treatment at all. "The tumor is probably benign," said the surgeon. "It's very reasonable to watch it closely with MRI scans and treat it only if it grows. It may stay this size for years."

Mark and his wife returned home, astounded yet pleased at having found this new option that they had not even considered before. Mark had overlooked this important option because his thinking was framed in terms of action. He had assumed that either surgery or chemotherapy would be essential, an assumption appealing to his aggressive style. Only when his frame shifted to a watch-and-wait strategy did he realize his full range of options.

If we are to identify all of our options, we must learn to think with different frames. We must think "outside the box."

Discover your frames.

HOW TO SHIFT FRAMES

Thinking of our options in terms of frames may seem abstract, and we might wonder if such mental effort is worthwhile. But surprisingly, the misuse of frames is one of the most common sources of poor decisions.

In their thoughtful book, *Decision Traps*, J. Edward Russo and Paul J.H. Schoemaker list the top ten most dangerous decision traps that have befuddled the fields of economics and business. Two of these ten relate directly to difficulties with frames. The time spent learning to manage frames is indeed worthwhile.

It is not easy to shift frames. Doing so requires that you challenge assumptions that you may barely know you have made. But there are some helpful tricks.

Try to think of all the reasons for and against your choice. Just as we did in the last section for our thoughts about the lottery, think of as many pros and cons as you can. Put some energy into this even if your mind is made up. If you favor surgery, list all the reasons you should *not* have surgery. These might include risk, recovery time, or loss of function. Be aggressive about attacking your position, because the goal is to use your discomfort to see things differently.

List your assumptions. You might believe surgery is quicker, or confers longer survival. List your assumptions and examine them carefully.

Ask a friend to play devil's advocate. Hearing our viewpoints challenged often opens our minds to new options.

Be on the lookout for frame shifts. You may have believed for years that taking vitamins serves no purpose, or you may have committed yourself to a long course of medical treatments. Then something happens—a phrase in an article, a comment from a friend, an internal voice—to suddenly change the way you look at vitamins or your treatments. Don't ignore these signals, and never think that it's too late to shift your thinking. Like shooting stars, opportunities for frame shifts are worth your attention even if they cannot be predicted.

List your goals, and make your lists as detailed as you can. Are you hoping for better control of your diabetes, or do you really want to be free of insulin? Do you want to survive your cancer as long as possible, or maintain a certain quality of life? Clearly stating our goals can sometimes highlight our assumptions and bring forth more options.

Examine what other people have done in your situation. What is obvious to others may be new to you.

All of this is hard work. You must be willing to consider different attitudes and keep an open mind. But the reward will be the discovery of new medical options that may make all the difference.

Think outside the frame.

SEARCH FOR DIFFICULT TRADEOFFS

Once you have identified the tradeoffs, don't allow yourself to focus on just those that make you feel content. Instead, concentrate on the really difficult ones. Concentrate on the tradeoffs that make you uncomfortable and for which there is no clear answer. The important issues are always the most disquieting.

Don't try to choose among your options at this point. The idea is not to come to a decision, but rather to prepare your mind by focusing on the crux of the problem. The actual decision will come more naturally at a later time. That such mental preparation is essential to inspire decisions has long been recognized. The famous physicist Helmholtz, for example, commented that his scientific inspirations "often enough crept quietly into my thinking without my suspecting their importance . . . in other cases they arrived suddenly, without any effort on my part . . . they liked especially to make their appearance while I was taking an easy walk over wooded hills in sunny weather!"

Insights come unexpectedly but inevitably to the prepared mind. Find the tradeoffs, understand the tough issues, and you're well on your way to a sound medical decision.

Savor the tough ones.

SEVEN

Step 3: Discovery of Data

Now we'll focus on the engine that drives all medical decisions: methods to gather reliable and meaningful medical data. We will start with some general preparations to make before beginning your search, and then show you how to use each source of medical information in detail.

—Preparing To Search—

It's Harder Than You Think

I have a confession to make. When I first began to write this book, I believed that finding medical information was a straightforward task. All you had to do was read the medical textbooks, search the Internet, talk with your doctors, and you would be done. You would then be ready to make your medical decision.

I wrote a detailed description of how to find and use the best medical books. I wrote elaborate instructions for finding good medical articles and for how to dissect them into small pieces that could be digested individually. I wrote about the nuances of medical writing and how to tell fact from controversy. I was encouraged that other medical authors were beginning to do the same and that more and more patients were using the Internet to find medical information.

But then I tried my own formula, applied to medical problems that I didn't know much about. And I failed. Badly.

The problem was that there were so many sources of medical information that I could not read them all. And worse, there were so many different opinions that I could not tell mainstream ideas accepted by everyone from more controversial viewpoints held by just a few. And I learned that my training in neurosurgery did not help at all.

To be sure, I think it is quite possible for anyone to gain a good perspective about any medical topic with some hard work and with time. But the time required might be more than you want to spend, especially if you are under the pressure of having to make decisions while ill.

I am not saying that you should give up your search for medical information. On the contrary, I believe that the more you search and dig and read, the better off you will be in making your medical decisions. What I am saying is that this process is harder than it appears, and that you will likely find it difficult to distinguish reliable medical thinking from more controversial opinions.

My goal in this chapter is to give you some tools that will make this difficult task easier. Do not be discouraged; doctors spend their entire lives learning to sift through medical information and still have difficulty finding all the relevant facts. Read, use your doctors as guides, and you will be rewarded with an understanding of your medical problems that will greatly enhance your medical decisions.

Medical literature is not easy.

REASONABLE EXPECTATIONS

Let's be clear about what you can and can't expect from your search through the medical literature.

Your efforts won't make you a medical expert. Doctors spend years and years to do this, and your time is more limited.

You won't understand everything you read. That's okay; you will get the gist of it. And even the experts don't understand everything.

You *can* broaden your medical knowledge about your problem. You'll understand your options much, much better if you read. This can only help you make better decisions.

You will be able to better discuss your treatment and diagnosis with your doctors. You will even be able to bring new ideas you have found to this discussion, ideas that may be of great benefit to both you and your doctor.

What I am telling you is not a popular or comforting viewpoint. We all hate to be told that it takes more than a little work to become an expert. But it's as true for medicine as it is for astrophysics or car repair.

Learn all you can within reason.

Do Your Homework

Have you ever wanted to design your dream house? Maybe you've imagined a large spiral staircase, or broad, floor-to-ceiling windows, or a real wine cellar. Perhaps you've already begun the rewarding task of building your personal castle.

But would you ever design your home without knowing something about insulation, drainage, and structural stability? Certainly not, although we usually rely on professionals for help with these technical topics. Still, most of us would try to learn something about basic house building before designing our homes.

The same is true for your medical decisions. Our goal, of course, is to solve our medical problems quickly. We need to decide for or against surgery, or which medication to take, as soon as possible. But just as in the case of building a house, a lot of background information is needed for our medical decisions. If we had all the time in the world, we would first learn about the human body, its nuances and diseases, before addressing our specific problems. We would learn how to build a house before designing our home.

But your time is not unlimited, and you will need to focus your efforts on your specific problem. Learning all of medicine first is not feasible; that is what your doctors are for. But I would encourage you to spend some time, however brief, to gather background information. If you have lung cancer, read a little about cancer in general. If you have sickle cell disease, learn a little about blood. Your efforts will pay off surprisingly quickly, and your background knowledge will enhance your decisions. After all, designing a home is easier and safer if you have an appreciation of the foundation.

Seek background.

MAKE SURE IT'S ABOUT YOU

Stephen Jay Gould was one of the most famous scientists of the twentieth century. An expert in evolution at Harvard University, he authored more than twenty books on evolutionary biology, wrote almost a thousand scientific articles, and was beloved for his colorful accounts of thorny scientific issues. He told a frightening story about his own health in an essay entitled, "The Median Isn't the Message."

Gould was found to have abdominal mesothelioma, a rare cancer that is usually rapidly fatal. When he learned his diagnosis after his surgery, he began to read about his tumor, discovering "with a gulp" that the median survival for those with this tumor was only eight months.

This news would be cause for despair for anyone, and Gould describes the next hour of his reading as furious and nervous. But what he found was that the eight-month limit did not apply directly to him. He was younger than those who died at eight months, and his cancer had been discovered at an earlier stage. And as Gould realized, statistics cannot ever predict what happens to the individual person.

Gould was right. And almost as if to prove it, he lived another twenty years after his discouraging diagnosis. Those grim estimates of mortality did not apply to people his age or at his stage of cancer. The statistics were not about him.

Human disease is a complex process. Small differences in the type of tumor, the patient's age at onset, or any of a multitude of factors can make enormous differences in the ultimate outcome. You will find, therefore, that medical writing is very specific. An article might address just one type of tumor, at a particular stage, in a particular group of patients. Or a study might look at the effects of a specific drug on a specific disease only in women of a certain age. Unless your circumstances exactly match the article, the conclusions might not be true for you.

Be careful to notice all these details. Make sure you are reading about your specific disease, your specific medications, applied to your own circumstances. Make sure that you are of the same age and gender as the patients studied, and that you have had the same treatments in the past. The details can make all the difference in the world.

It has to be you.

SEEK PAINFUL INFORMATION

Which would you rather daydream about: a three-week trip to Tahiti or your income tax return?

If you chose your tax return, you can skip this section. Otherwise, read on.

It's only natural to dwell on pleasant topics and avoid painful ones. This preference is strong and extends to more than daydreams. Psychologists know, for example, that most of us believe we will enjoy good health and financial success in the future, even though the statistics show that this cannot be true for everyone. And we would even rather look at images of happiness than images of sadness. One scientific study illustrated this fact by finding that people had more difficulty remembering a frowning face than a smiling face. Our preference for pleasant runs deep.

The same is true when we consider our medical problems. We will pay more attention to research promising pleasant outcomes than to studies predicting our death and morbidity. A patient with cancer may seize upon a report of a successful treatment, ignoring other research that does not support such a rosy result.

The flip side of this behavior is also common; predictions of death and doom are often remembered with stark clarity. The impact of even a single report of one patient suffering a gloomy end can be devastating to the concerned reader, overpowering the impact of more complete studies in which the outcomes are pleasant.

Nobody can make you like unpleasantness. But the most useful and honest medical information is often the most frightening. We must therefore make a conscious effort to seek out the most disturbing information when we are making our medical decisions, momentarily suppressing our natural tendency to see only the good and the pleasant. Only in this way will we be able to see all the possibilities.

Seek the unpleasant.

ALL SOURCES HAVE AN AGENDA

Information reaches us through people. The stories we read in the newspaper are written by people, as are the facts we find in books and the medical information we discover in the course of our research. Only rarely do we uncover a snippet of information in pure form, untouched by human hands or minds.

This means that every anecdote, every story, and every report that we read is told to us through the eyes of another. And always, the viewpoints and perceptions of that other person creep into the story alongside the bare facts. It is an unavoidable aspect of human communication: No story can be told apart from the storyteller.

I will use the word *agenda* to refer to these viewpoints behind the stories, as well as the motivation and subjective assumptions of the storyteller. All human beings have agendas, and all human communication is colored by their presence.

While some agendas are benign or accidental, others are rather deliberate. Advertisements are the most obvious examples, the agenda being to sell you the chosen product whether you really need it or not. Newspaper articles have agendas, even while striving to be unbiased. After all, every reporter feels pressure to make a story seem interesting so that the paper will sell. And there are always political and ideological biases of both the reporter and the editor.

Let me share a secret with you: Medical literature is no exception. Certainly, medical advertisements are no less deliberate than any other advertisement. And newspaper articles about medical topics can be just as biased as other newspaper articles. But even scientific medical articles are often molded by agendas that may not be obvious. The author may have invested his or her career in a certain treatment and may be defending or promoting that treatment with the article. The research behind an article on a particular medication might be funded by a drug company, and we can only guess what prejudices might be hidden. The author may be embroiled in a controversy with a colleague, so that the conclusions of the article are written more to make a point than to provide a balanced perspective. Medical literature is not innocent.

Medical textbooks are probably less affected by agendas than other sources. I suspect this is because the authors are generally poorly paid (if they are paid at all), so that monetary reward does not determine what they choose to write. Instead, they are motivated by their desire to become respected authorities and to acquire an eminent position within the medical community. Their reputation grows if the textbook becomes an authoritative reference, so that these books tend to be grounded in fact and written with balanced perspective.

But make no mistake, every source of information carries the agenda of its creator, the assumptions and subjective viewpoints of its author. It is therefore worthwhile to try to imagine what these agendas might be, and in so doing to continue cultivating skepticism, as I advised earlier. The idea is not to discard those sources in which you detect an agenda, but to use your knowledge to more properly judge the information contained in their pages.

Keep an eye on the agenda.

NOBODY TELLS IT STRAIGHT

We often rely on others to tell us what is really true, asking those around us to "Tell it to me straight." While we do not expect a reasonable reply from car salesmen, we often ask the absolute truth from our good friends, close family, and physicians. "The straight truth" is one of the few sources of information that we would trust with our lives.

But "the straight truth" doesn't really exist.

No one can tell a story, or relate a fact, or impart information with complete objectivity. We all have viewpoints and assumptions that determine how we tell our stories. The very act of choosing which facts to tell introduces the subjective thoughts and choices of the narrator.

Even our nightly newscasts, reporting the bare facts of news, will be interpreted differently if the announcer is grim and terse rather than relaxed and smiling.

Here is an example that is as incredible as it is disturbing. A multi-institutional group of scientists headed by social psychologist Brian Mullen at Syracuse University studied the network news coverage of the 1984 presidential election, focusing their attention on the question of whether *how* the news was delivered could change the *perception* of the news by the viewer. They found that the facial expressions exhibited by the newscasters—subtle cues we rely upon for nonverbal communication—could depend upon what the newscaster was talking about. In particular, they found that the facial expressions of ABC's anchor Peter Jennings were more positive when he was discussing Ronald Reagan than when he was discussing the other candidates. More astonishing, they found that viewers who watched Peter Jennings were more likely to have voted for Ronald Reagan. In other words, even the most professional, dispassionate sources of information can contain unconscious hints that dramatically affect our interpretation.

Physicians are no exception to these influences, even while talking with you about your medical options. It is simply impossible to present different aspects of any issue completely objectively because such perfect objectivity does not exist. A slip of intonation, a dropped vowel, the way the doctor sits in the chair or makes eye contact—you will hear all of these subtle cues as loudly as if they were screamed into a megaphone. This happens at an unconscious level, through the subtle sensitivities that are so well developed in humans. Our bodies show our viewpoints to others, even as we try so hard to be objective.

I am not considering extreme cases in which the doctor makes a conscious attempt to sway the patient one way or the other, but rather, those more frequent times when the physician is really trying to eliminate bias. It can't be done.

Consider this example: Suppose your physicians have discovered that you have a heart condition that could lead to disabling fatigue and shortness of breath. Suppose also that there is an operation that could prevent this from happening, but that it is a major operation with potential complications. Here are two ways to tell you the news:

Explanation 1: "Without this operation, your breathing could get so bad that you could die."

Explanation 2: "The operation may or may not protect you against any further damage to your heart."

These two explanations are based on the same information, but convey dramatically different messages. Which explanation would move you toward having the surgery?

This does not mean you must distrust everyone and listen to no one. Just be aware that no one can tell you the absolute truth, the ultimate straight scoop, on any medical topic. No physician has all the answers, although many can be very useful to you in your search for good decisions. Talk to lots of people; read as much as you can; form your own opinions. The absolute truth is simply not available from any one person.

Know the author's agenda.

—THE SOURCES—

Having reviewed our expectations and cultivated our skepticism, it is now time to go and get the data. This section will show you how to effectively use each of the many sources of medical data.

BOOKS

MEDICAL BOOKS

We live in the age of the computer, of gigabyte hard disks and high-speed Internet connections. Information flies past us from thousands of Web sites containing millions of topics without end. And yet my favorite source for medical information is still the book.

But not all books, since not all medical books are equally helpful. Some are quite specialized, written for experts and outdated as soon as they are published. Others emphasize a particular technique or skill, such as interpreting ultrasound studies, that usually is not needed by those making medical decisions. And others are simply poorly written, a feature all too common to many fields of study.

The books that will be most helpful to us are medical textbooks. These books are truly giants, as intimidating in their scope as they are difficult to carry in both arms. The topic of each is clearly defined by its title, usually a well-defined but large chunk of medicine: internal medicine, surgery, pediatrics, or obstetrics ("internal medicine" usually means general medicine). Their length typically runs into the thousands of pages, requiring the combined writing efforts of tens or even hundreds of authors. They serve the medical community as the main repositories of medical knowledge, consulted by experts and students alike. We need to be able to use them, too, and you will be pleased to hear that, with a little work, they are quite usable.

Medical textbooks are my favorite source of information not only because of their content, but because they are enduringly reliable. The reason is surprising: No one makes a lot of money by writing a medical book. The demand for medical books is relatively small, limited to medical libraries and doctors. Profits from sales are correspondingly small, so that the motivation for writing these books cannot be a wish for financial gain or a desire to entertain. Rather, they are written to create a useful source of information or to establish the authors or editors as authorities. Luckily for us, this means that the medical textbook is an unusually balanced and complete source of medical information.

I also favor medical textbooks because they are a great source of background information. Just as a background knowledge of the general plan of a large city's streets will help us find our destination, so will a small amount of background medical knowledge permit us to find our way to a useful decision. We touched on the importance of obtaining background knowledge earlier in this book, and medical textbooks provide that very important opportunity.

I must confess to some personal reasons I prefer medical textbooks. I enjoy the feel and heft of a real book, its fonts and binding. And my enjoyment of physically leafing through a book may have something to do with the fact that I am better at retrieving information from books than from electronic sources. Another reason is that books give up all their information at once, unlike the stingy Internet, which divvies out one page of information at a time. But regardless of these quirky personal preferences, the modern medical textbook is a godsend to those seeking medical information and should not be forgotten even as we plug in to the Internet.

There are some disadvantages to medical books. Because books take some time to publish, you will not find the very latest medical information in a textbook. You will have to supplement your search with medical articles if you want the latest and greatest. Medical books can also be intimidating, in both their length and their language. It may seem difficult to locate what you need within the thousands of written pages, and then it may seem difficult to understand what you find.

But medical textbooks contain both the specific facts and the general background you need for your medical decisions. They are meant to be read and used by real people. Armed with a few tricks, your efforts will be rewarded a thousandfold.

Nothing beats a book.

How to Use a Medical Textbook

The first step in using a medical textbook is to find the book itself, since most are not carried by your local bookstore. Nor would you necessarily buy one if you found it there, since the price can approach that of a small car. The easiest place to find medical textbooks is in the medical libraries of large medical schools. These libraries will usually allow you to use their books while you are there, but won't usually allow you to take the books home. (A list of medical schools in this country can be found at www.aamc.org.) The librarians are typically both knowledgeable and helpful, and can rapidly guide you to the standard medical textbooks. You can also find medical textbooks in medical bookstores, but, again, the price is usually steep and the selection limited when compared with a library. A third source is your doctor, who may allow you to use his or her own medical textbooks in the office.

Once you've found your book, make sure you have the correct subject. If you have lung cancer, don't read a book on obstetrics. If your child is ill, start with a textbook of pediatrics. And because many illnesses can be treated with medications or surgery, you may want to consult textbooks of both medicine and surgery.

Let's start with the example of lung cancer. Since cancer is frequently treated with medications, we turn to a medical textbook as the best source of general information. We can look in surgical textbooks later if we need more detailed surgical information.

Our medical textbook is made of two volumes housing an intimidating three thousand pages. The best place to start is the Table of Contents, which is itself as long as a small book. We will look for a specific mention of lung cancer rather than more general discussions of cancer and its treatment, since each of the chapters can be hundreds of pages long and we want to be efficient in our search. You may find several chapters on lung cancer, perhaps one each for general discussion, diagnosis, and treatment.

The book index may be helpful, especially if your topic is highly specific. Be aware that these indices are exhaustive, and that it may take time to look at all the indicated pages.

Once you have found your chapters, skim them first to see what is there. It is likely that you will not want to concentrate on every detail on first reading, and some portions might require you to do some background reading elsewhere. Discussions of illness involving the liver, for example, often begin with an introduction to the complex topic of liver physiology. You may wish to skip this at first and return if needed.

As you begin your reading, be aware that you will not understand everything you find. But because medical textbooks are written to be used, you will probably be pleased to find yourself quickly learning the important facts. In the case of lung cancer, you will find that there are two major types, called small-cell and non–small-cell lung cancer, each with its own prognosis and preferred treatment. One is best treated with surgery, the other with chemotherapy. Exactly what a "small cell" is may not be exactly clear, but no matter; you have learned something important about lung cancer that will help you both to understand your doctor and to make better decisions.

You may wish to have a medical dictionary handy as you read your chapters, although I would advise you not to go overboard with its use. Look up the words you need for understanding, but accept that it may take a second or third reading to absorb everything. It is more important at this stage to get the major points than to get bogged down with every word.

As you gather your information, take as many notes as you need to remember the key points. Bring plenty of paper, because there will be a lot of information. You may also want to make copies of the important chapters, and most libraries will have copying machines available for a reasonable fee. This will permit you to reread the chapter later at your leisure, and is often well worth the effort.

Medical textbooks are not written to comfort you as a patient. They are handbooks for doctors in which no punches are pulled. You will therefore find estimates of prognosis given rather harshly as percentages, and stark descriptions of diseases that may afflict you in the future. Although a frank discussion of your medical problem can be invaluable to your plans, it is never pleasant to read a description of your future demise. But this unpleasantness is one of the prices you must pay for admittance into these medical storehouses of knowledge. Take heart, however, if what you read seems gloomy. You are not a statistic, your circumstances are not completely average, and medical textbooks are always a bit out of date—remember what we said about Stephan Jay Gould. Keep reading and talking with your doctors for more accurate estimates of your future.

Don't be intimidated; medical textbooks are written to be used.

REFERENCE BOOKS

A number of helpful books in common use are not quite medical textbooks, but are nevertheless reliable and at times essential. These include medical dictionaries as well as the *Physician's Desk Reference*, which contains thorough descriptions of prescription drugs and their side effects. Other reference books such as the *Merck Manual* are updated yearly to address newer topics.

These books and others are listed along with a brief description below.

A WARNING

One last word to the wise. Hundreds of books about medicine and health are written every year and there is no accepted universal rating system. Some of these are incomplete and poorly written, while others are frank deceptions aimed directly at the medical consumer (that's you).

Caveat emptor: Buyer beware.

SUGGESTED MEDICAL TEXTBOOKS AND REFERENCE BOOKS

Here are a few samples of the many medical textbooks in common use. This list is by no means complete, and I have omitted some topics, such as emergency medicine, that may be less relevant for those making medical decisions. Be aware that standard textbooks exist for every conceivable medical issue and that your librarian can guide you to the many fine textbooks that space does not permit me to include. I will include the first author or editor and publisher but not the entire reference for each.

General Texts: Medicine and Surgery

You will probably consult these first, moving on to more specialized texts if needed.

Harrison's Principles of Internal Medicine (E. Braunwald, editor; McGraw-Hill). This has been a standard text for many years, similar to the one used in our lung cancer example in the last section, and is an excellent source for general medicine. It is no longer written by Harrison (modern texts now require many authors), although it still carries his name. This is a good place to start your search.

Cecil Textbook of Medicine (L. Goldman, editor; W.B. Saunders). Another well-respected and standard classic text of medicine. The articles are clear and relevant, and this book is a great place to start your search.

Kelley's Textbook of Internal Medicine (H.D. Humes, editor; Lippincott, Williams & Wilkins). A third large textbook of medicine.

Principles of Surgery (S.I. Schwartz, editor; McGraw-Hill). A classic and complete textbook of surgery and surgical diseases, with chapters on general surgical issues as well as specific operations. Most of the time you should also consult a general medicine textbook to learn the non-surgical viewpoint.

Sabiston Textbook of Surgery (C.M. Townsend, editor; W.B. Saunders). Another classic textbook of general surgery, also huge in scope.

Rudolph's Pediatrics (C.D. Rudolph, editor; McGraw-Hill). A standard textbook of diseases of babies, infants, and children. Medicine for children is often so different from medicine for adults that consultation with a pediatrics text is a must if the patient is young.

Specific Diseases and Disorders

Cancer Medicine (R.C. Bast, American Cancer Society, B.C. Decker). Most of the time, a general textbook on internal medicine or surgery will contain all you need to know (or want to know) about cancer. This somewhat technical but complete volume will give you more details about all aspects of cancer and its treatment.

Cancer. Principles and Practice of Oncology (V.T. DeVita, editor; Lippincott, Williams & Wilkins). This two-volume work is another excellent supplement to your reading about cancer. It is complete and yet quite readable.

Textbook of Critical Care (A. Grenvik, editor; W.B. Saunders). This large text covers the intricate and specialized treatment given in the modern intensive care unit. In most cases, you will want to consult a general medicine or surgery text before taking on this specialized text, but its chapters can be useful for those with loved ones being treated in "the unit."

Williams Obstetrics (F.G. Cunningham, editor; McGraw-Hill). A standard textbook of obstetrics, addressing the normal birth as well as everything that can go wrong.

Novak's Gynecology (J.S. Berek, editor; Lippincott, Williams & Wilkins). A very readable account of gynecologic diseases and their treatment (obstetrics not included).

Principles of Neurology (M. Victor, editor; McGraw-Hill). The description of neurological diseases such as multiple sclerosis and Parkinson's disease is so specialized and extensive that a large and readable text such as this is a welcome and even an essential extension of the general medicine texts. Be aware that many rare disorders are described, and you may want to stick with the main topics. The explanations are clear and relevant.

Textbook of Clinical Psychiatry (R.E. Hales, editor; American Psychiatric Publishing). A readable standard textbook of psychiatric disease.

Kaplan & Sadock's Comprehensive Textbook of Psychiatry (B.J. Sadock, editor; Lippincott, Williams & Wilkins). A two-volume, complete text of psychiatric disease.

Campbell's Operative Orthopedics (S.T. Canale, editor; Mosby). A standard but large (four volumes) text describing all manner of fractures and orthopedic injuries and their treatment.

Surgery of the Chest (D.C. Sabiston, editor; W.B. Saunders). Most of the time you will consult a general textbook of surgery to learn about these specialized operations, but this is a good standard text if you want more.

Campbell's Urology (P.C. Walsh, editor; W.B. Saunders). This four-volume text contains everything you might want to know about urologic diseases. Again, you will probably start with a general surgery text first.

Blood. Principles and Practice of Hematology (R.I. Handin, editor; J.B. Lippincott). A full treatment of a specialized topic, everything from anemia to leukemia. Use this if you need more than a general medicine textbook.

Endocrinology (L.J. DeGroot, editor; W.B. Saunders). A three-volume text addressing the specialized field of endocrinology (glands and hormones). Use a general medical textbook first.

Encyclopedia of Human Nutrition (M.J. Sadler, editor; Academic Press). This three-volume text is an exhaustive treatment of nutrition and its relation to disease. Included is everything from fatty acids to gout to zinc; use this for all your questions about nutrition and medicine.

Metabolic and Molecular Bases of Inherited Disease (C.R. Scriver, editor; McGraw-Hill). This four-volume text is specialized indeed, for it focuses on rare inherited diseases that usually receive skimpy treatment in general textbooks. Once you know you are dealing with one of these unusual disorders, this book can be informative when other sources are silent.

Reference Works

These books are designed to be used as needed rather than read from cover to cover. They can give you vital supplemental information, adding to your understanding of the medical issues.

Gray's Anatomy (Churchill Livingstone). This huge volume has been the complete and standard reference work on human anatomy for almost 150 years and represents a marvel of civilization: a description and illustration of every anatomical aspect of the human body. You wouldn't want to read this from cover to cover—the details are occasionally burdensome, and other texts may be more readable—but this is the horse's mouth for anatomy.

Atlas of Human Anatomy (F. Netter, Novartis). This is a gorgeous work, as are all the illustrations of the renowned medical artist, Frank Netter. His drawings are not only crystal clear and informative, but they are beautiful works of art that are a pleasure to study. If a picture is worth a thousand words, each of these is easily worth a million. Five minutes' perusal of these could save you an hour of anatomical reading.

A Regional Atlas of the Human Body (C. Clemente, editor; Williams & Wilkins). This atlas also combines informative anatomy with beautiful illustrations, sometimes in more graphic detail than Netter's atlas. Don't skip this if you see it on the shelf.

Goodman and Gilman's Pharmacological Basis of Therapeutics (J.G. Hardman, editor; McGraw-Hill). Its long and intricate name is appropriate for this long and intricate book, which is a well-respected reference. In it you will find an exhaustive treatment of medications and how they work. It is tough going, and you may want to consult the PDR (see below) or one of the many practical handbooks about drugs, but this is the source for details and mechanisms.

Physician's Desk Reference ("The PDR") (Medical Economics Co.). This contains brief if not terse descriptions of every prescription drug on the American market, describing uses, doses, and toxicity. This source is used by every doctor and nurse. The order is not alphabetic, so use the index pages found in the middle of the book. Nonprescription drugs are covered in a separate edition of the PDR.

Merck Manual of Diagnosis and Therapeutics (Merck Research Laboratories). This small but thick encyclopedia contains beautifully worded descriptions of a host of diseases and their treatments. You will find a blend of medical and surgical issues here, befitting the book's role as a handbook for practicing physicians. A reference worth knowing about.

Washington Manual of Ambulatory Therapeutics (T.L. Lin; Lippincott, Williams & Wilkins). This spiral-bound volume gives you a bird's-eye view of general medicine from a practical standpoint. How-to topics include prescribing intravenous solutions and choosing antibiotics. Meant as a handbook for practicing physicians, its telegraphic style and nuts-and-bolts detail may not be relevant to your needs, but it is a good source for descriptions of how to treat disease.

Dorland's Illustrated Medical Dictionary (W.B. Saunders). This is one of many fine medical dictionaries and has been a standard for many years. The inclusion of illustrations is a nice feature adding to the clear explanations.

Taber's Cyclopedic Medical Dictionary (F.A. Davis) and *Stedman's Medical Dictionary* (Williams & Wilkins). Two more standard medical dictionaries of high quality.

Books are your friends.

ARTICLES

MEDICAL ARTICLES

Medical textbooks are wonderful sources of information, but because of the time taken for publication, they are never up-to-date. Doctors and researchers instead publish their most current results in one of several hundred professional medical journals. These magazines are usually monthlies and contain articles aimed at the working expert. But they are valuable sources for us as well, frequently summarizing the latest modern concepts of treatment and revealing the newest results. Known as "the literature," this massive collection of articles is frequently difficult to use but just as frequently contains gems of medical writing and information.

But why should you bother to struggle with these technical works? They are not written for the general public and they make no attempt to be easily readable or even balanced in presentation. In fact, you may choose not to bother with medical articles at all, sticking instead to medical books and discussions with your doctors. But many people want more information or the latest options that may not be widely known, and the Internet gives them the ready access to "the literature" that they crave. With a little patience, your efforts can be rewarded a hundredfold, so I have included some detailed advice about how to find and interpret good medical articles.

I want to make a distinction between medical journals that are peer-reviewed and those that are not. A journal is "peer-reviewed" if every article in that journal has been read thoroughly and approved by one or more experts in the field prior to publication. These expert reviewers are expected to be highly critical of a potential article, maintaining high standards as well as high rejection rates. The peer-review process has its faults, but is generally a good method of ensuring quality.

Most journals that you will find in a medical library are peer-reviewed, and I would be skeptical of journals that are not. You can determine whether the journal you are using is peer-reviewed by looking at its fine print in the first few pages or by asking the librarian.

Unlike medical textbooks, *medical articles* are often narrowly focused, frequently biased, and often filled with controversy. An author may present data supporting a peculiar aspect of treatment, or wish to support a favorite but controversial theory. A particular viewpoint or unusual technique might be presented without discussion of more conventional treatment, and the importance (or lack thereof) of the article might be impossible to determine for those who are not experts in the field. In either case, the article might be misleading to those without a hefty amount of background. Again, caveat emptor.

Some medical articles are *review articles*, written to summarize the latest thinking about a disease or its treatment. For example, you may find an article reviewing the rationale for different treatments of fractures of the elbow. Such an article may discuss the pros and cons of the different treatments and therefore be of far greater value than a technical article reporting the merits of only one particular new treatment. Most reviews are well written and complete, although the quality is not as uniform as it is for book chapters. These articles are nevertheless worth finding and reading. (We'll address finding review articles on the Internet later on.)

Another type of medical article is the *clinical series*. This report documents the effects of the treatment in question on a large number of patients. The idea is that since the treatment works for so many people, it must be worthwhile. In fact, some doctors will not accept a medical statement as fact unless it has been proven with a clinical series.

Distinct from a clinical series is the *case report*. This is an anecdotal account of only one patient, written to demonstrate a novel treatment or a new disease. Most doctors do not consider case reports to be proof of anything; they are more like testimonials (which we will discuss later). But case reports are worthwhile because they illustrate valuable or provocative ideas.

So what can we realistically hope to obtain from medical articles? We can hope to find the latest in medical thinking and treatment. We can hope to find discussions of medical controversy and reviews of background medical information. And we can hope to find a whole lot of new and different ideas.

The disadvantage of the "medical literature" is that it is much like a collection of works in progress; you cannot believe everything you read. Today's new idea may be proven false tomorrow, and it is difficult to find the one right answer in the midst of controversy. It is therefore best to remain skeptical and demand that a treatment be proven in several articles before you surrender your trust.

Medical articles are works in progress.

HOW TO READ A MEDICAL ARTICLE

Before you can read anything, you have to find the article first.

Find a top-quality article that is relevant to your needs. This is not a trivial task, since there are literally millions of articles to choose from and thousands appear every day. Try to focus on articles that are relevant to the difficulties you are having with your decisions. This means that you will be focusing on articles that address the options and trade-offs you have found for yourself, as we discussed in the first steps of making medical decisions.

The best way to find medical articles is to search the Internet, and we will show you in detail how to do this a little later in this chapter. The articles listed at the end of book chapters can also be useful, although the chapters themselves usually contain the pertinent information in the article itself.

Check who wrote the article and when it was written. Data from a renowned cancer center or publication in a prestigious medical journal may be particularly compelling, although this is not an ironclad guarantee of high quality. Articles published more than five years ago may already be out of date.

Realize that you will not understand everything you read. This is not an insult; even most experts will not understand every detail, and I can assure you that I do not understand everything I read outside of my own specialty. But it is quite possible to extract a great deal of useful information from these articles, and to extract all of it if you have the time. Use a dictionary as needed, make copies of the best articles to read over later, and don't forget to talk with your doctors.

Understand the organization of the article. Most medical articles are organized in a very particular fashion. They begin with a terse summary of the article, called an *Abstract*, which is typically only a few paragraphs long. Following that is an *Introduction*, in which the author states the problem addressed by the article. Then there is a *Methods* section, in which details of the experimental methods are laid out. These are important details that can be difficult for the nonexpert. The data are then presented in the *Results* section, often as a dry recitation of numbers. Finally, and most important, the article ends with a *Discussion* section, in which the author summarizes data, attacks or supports other theories, and argues for the final conclusions.

There are as many ways of reading a medical article as there are of cooking an apple pie, but I will show you my approach. Let's consider as an example an article comparing two types of chemotherapy for breast cancer. I first skim the *Abstract*, hoping to get the general flavor of the article. The *Abstract* is organized as a mini-article, containing paragraphs summarizing the *Introduction*, *Methods*, *Results*, and *Conclusion* (rather than *Discussion*) sections. Here we will find a brief statement of the importance of the two types of chemotherapy, a quick summary of how the study was conducted and the raw results, and a paragraph stating the preferred conclusions of the authors. I often focus on the

Introduction and *Conclusion* sections, since the entire *Abstract* is curt and usually difficult to understand on the first reading.

I then read the *Introduction* section of the article, slowly if necessary. Here we find out why the two chemotherapeutic agents are important, and why we might want to compare them. Perhaps one has unfortunate side effects but the other has not been proven effective. I will then skim the *Methods* and *Results* section, hoping to gain a sense of what was studied and how. We will have to return to these sections later if we really want to understand the article, but they are difficult and can be scanned in the beginning.

I then read the *Discussion* section carefully, for it is here that the conclusions and implications of the article are found. The author will summarize the data and argue for certain interpretations. In our example, we might find that one drug is far better and safer than the other. Work by previous researchers is usually summarized and sometimes criticized. And a discussion of the implications of the work is usually included along with the author's recommendations. We might find, for example, a suggestion that a specific type of chemotherapy should be used for certain stages of breast cancer.

At this point, we must decide whether to read the article again, this time more carefully. We have discovered what the article is about and read its conclusions, but we do not have enough information to evaluate the article. If the conclusions are interesting, and if we think the article is worthwhile, the next step is to read the *Methods* and *Results* section more carefully to fill in the gaps.

The *Methods* section is the most treacherous part of the article. Here you will find a rather bland recitation of which patients were studied, which treatments were compared, which diagnostic tests were used, what the authors meant by success and failure, and how the statistics were interpreted. Medical scientists spend their entire careers learning to distinguish good methods from bad, and are still sometimes fooled. On occasion a well-known article will be declared invalid years later, only because of a new and subtle analysis of its methods.

The *Results* section is just that: a list of results from each part of the study. Sometimes the author includes interpretive remarks to aid your thinking, while at other times the list is fairly dry. It is easy to get lost in the detail here, but try to find the major results important to you. In our example of the two chemotherapeutic agents, try to find which drug produced the longest or most frequent remission, and which drug produced the worst complications. Be aware that the author is trying to quantify results in as many ways as possible, frequently causing us more than a little confusion.

Results are often given as percentages and averages, along with an estimate of error (the "standard deviation"). There are a number of tools that will help you to interpret this data, tools that I will discuss in detail in chapter eight.

Here I wish to make two points. First, make sure the study is relevant to you. If patients with advanced breast cancer are being studied but you have early breast cancer, chances are the conclusions of the study will not be true for you. Second, analysis of *Methods* and *Results* is tricky business. Don't be shy about enlisting the help of your own local expert, your doctor.

Finally, read the *Abstract* again, this time carefully. This summary will review the article for you, occasionally with an emphasis you may have missed in the first reading. Read the entire article as many times as you think necessary if the article seems to be important. Use our techniques of analysis given in chapters eight and nine, consult your doctors, and you will have extracted what you need to know.

Articles are worth the effort.

PRACTICE GUIDELINES

Doctors have been pressured in recent years to create and provide standardized guidelines for the treatment of nearly every illness. Part of this pressure comes from the realization that high-quality medicine is not practiced everywhere, and that written guidelines could improve this sad state of affairs. More pressure comes from insurance companies and HMOs, agencies needing common standards to construct responsible financial plans.

In response to these pressures, professional medical groups such as the American Medical Association have written and published lists of recommendations known as *practice guidelines*. These are lists of preferred treatments and ways to diagnose a variety of diseases, arrived at by a consensus of experts. They are not collected in any one journal or book, but you will find them from time to time in your reading.

Practice guidelines can be useful in our search for good decisions, for they summarize what experts believe to be important in the management of a particular illness. You may think of new ideas when you read these recommendations, or formulate a new starting point for discussions with your doctor. However, be aware that the use of practice guidelines is not without problems.

First, critics would point out that because medicine is an art rather than a science, no list of guidelines can capture what is just right for you. It is wrong, therefore, to take guidelines as the final word for your medical care.

Second, guidelines have been used to justify choices based on cost rather than quality, especially if the guidelines are formulated by an insurance company or HMO.

Third, there is no way to know how good a particular set of guidelines really is; there are no guidelines for guidelines.

Finally, guidelines rapidly become outdated. A recent report from RAND, reported in the *Journal of the American Medical Association*, found that more than three-quarters of the guidelines published by the U.S. Agency for Healthcare Research and Quality were obsolete.

As you come across practice guidelines, make careful note of them and discuss them with your doctors. They can be useful organizers of your thoughts and perhaps springboards to new ideas. But be aware that their origins might be political or financial, and that no general scheme can apply perfectly to each individual.

Guidelines are not written in stone.

NEWSLETTERS, NEWSPAPERS, TELEVISION, AND ADVERTISEMENTS

It may seem odd that I group these four sources together, since they are all so different from one another. Newsletters are brief summaries of items of medical interest, frequently circulated by medical groups or medical companies. Newspapers contain reports of medical events that must remain factual if the readership is to remain faithful. Television, of course, presents medical information in many different ways. Documentaries, talk shows, and newscasts report factual information, much like a newspaper. But there are also fictionalized depictions of hospitals and doctors, exposing millions of viewers to medical ideas and medical practice. Finally, advertisements of medical products and services are all too common no matter where we look.

I group these disparate sources together because they share one common fact: You cannot believe a word they say.

More precisely, I believe that you cannot distinguish medical fact from fallacy within these sources. Let me explain this controversial opinion.

Medical newsletters. These brief summaries of medical topics are distributed by a variety of organizations. Some newsletters are written by experts and accepted by most medical authorities. Others are thinly veiled advertisements for certain drugs or equipment, written by an agent for the pharmaceutical company or manufacturer. More insidiously, some newsletters claim legitimacy from the inclusion of well-known experts, but in fact are biased toward a particular drug or service. The point is that these articles are not peer reviewed and are not subject to a responsible editorial board. Some are very good, some are very bad, and most are in between. Unless you are an insider, it is difficult to know which is which.

Newspapers. Newspapers are more reliable, since their continued existence depends on the credibility of their reports. But there are still problems. Both the reporter and the editor may feel pressure to make their report seem more interesting or positive than it deserves to be. The necessary brevity of a newspaper story can hide important aspects of medical events. Errors sometimes creep in, confusing even the careful reader. And newspapers themselves are occasionally fooled by flimflam artists. The result: The information you find in newspapers cannot always be taken as gospel.

Television. TV is not much better. Someone once described television as a series of commercials separated by programming designed to keep us from changing the channel. To keep us away from the channel changer, television must show us a constantly changing cavalcade of energy and entertainment. And it must be simple and quick, lacking any of the time-consuming details that would add substance to the story. Any reports of medical events in this hurried atmosphere should therefore be taken with a grain of salt, and sometimes with the whole saltshaker. There simply cannot be a new "medical breakthrough" every week, as the hype of television would have us believe.

To be sure, medical issues are usually covered responsibly on television, and in fact, some people trust these reports as much as they trust their own doctor. My wife, for example, is one of millions of viewers who has formed a "television relationship" with a popular talk-show host, absolutely trusting her medical reporting. And with good reason, since the reports on that show are accurate and responsible. But on the next channel you can find accounts of the effects of moonbeams on heart disease and infomercials on the merits of the latest exercise device. Sober and responsible reporting exists side by side with nonsense, and sometimes you can't tell them apart.

An unexpected feature of television is how well medical issues and ideas can be depicted by completely fictitious drama. The drama series *ER*, for example, often demonstrates the medical practice of an emergency room more vividly and accurately than could any documentary or news report. So don't ignore television dramas; it is quite conceivable that these shows could serve as a fruitful starting point for further research into the medical literature and discussions with your doctor.

Advertisements. No one considers ads to be unbiased sources of information. But like it or not, we obtain part of our medical information from advertising. We are made aware of new drugs available to treat hair loss, surgery for impaired vision, and vitamins for any condition that ails us. And who can watch TV for more than a few minutes without being forced to hear about the hygienic benefits of some new mouthwash?

What all these sources have in common is that they cannot be taken at face value. Whether they are composed of true facts or complete fiction, they must be investigated further before we can trust them as medical truth. But these sources can be wonderful generators of new ideas, alerting us to possibilities that we would have overlooked otherwise. It doesn't matter that you've learned about a new treatment for cancer in the newspaper or on *ER*; what matters is that you have learned about it and that you have the opportunity to investigate further. True, I am a believer in the mundane tools of medical literature and discussion with doctors. But we must not throw away any information bestowed upon us by our irrational and accidental world.

Use everything you've got.

THE INTERNET

In a popular television commercial, a well-dressed businesswoman is demonstrating a computer feature to a vast audience of other business people. The feature is this: Click on a word on your computer screen, and another screen will instantly pop up with information on the topic described by that word. No more searches! Immediate and convenient knowledge about anything you like! The crowd likes it a little, then a lot, then starts chanting and raving about the imagined prospects.

But who decides what information we get? And—more important—what information we *don't* get?

This vignette summarizes the power and problem of the Internet. It is a tool of unimaginable connectivity, of access to information at speeds we once thought impossible. But it is also a wild, human creation, full of solid truth and outright lies and everything in between. It is too powerful a tool for us to ignore when we seek medical information, and yet it is a double-edged tool that can cause injury if not used carefully. In this section, we will discuss some ways to use the Internet safely.

The American public discovered the Internet for medical use a long time ago. The Pew Internet and American Life Project reports that 55 million Americans used the Internet in 2000 to obtain medical information, and that most of these people continue to use it for that purpose at least once a month. A full 70% of these 55 million Americans reported that their medical decisions had been influenced by what they learned on the Internet. And most Americans trust the Internet, as 64% of us will use a medical Web site without knowing anything about it.

We all know theoretically that the Internet contains garbage as well as gems, junk intermixed with pearls. What may not be as obvious is that the garbage can be dressed up to look like jewelry, using any number of inexpensive Web site software tools to produce a sophisticated appearance with a minimum of effort. And there is always the specter of bias. How far would you trust a Web site sponsored by a pharmaceutical company to tell you about their competitor's medications?

But is the Internet really all that bad? Those who distribute medical information must surely feel an ethical and legal obligation to be accurate. Can't we at least trust the medical Web sites?

Apparently not. Like other aspects of the Web, there is absolutely no regulation of the content of medical Web sites. Attempts to do this with voluntary sets of rules such as the HON (Health on the Net) Code are flawed, because medical Web sites are not required to comply and these codes involve self-assessment. And it gets worse. The Federal Trade Commission estimates that about half of the medical content put on the Web is never even reviewed by a doctor.

Medical Web sites were recently studied by Gretchen K. Berland and her colleagues at several academic institutions in California. Their findings, published in the *Journal of the American Medical Association* (a peer-reviewed journal, of course), summarize the quality of information found on medical Web sites as well as their ease of use. The overall report card was dismal.

Berland's group studied the ability of fourteen major search engines and twenty-five major medical Web sites to provide information about four topics: breast cancer, depression, obesity, and childhood asthma. They found that only 20% of the first pages of each search contained anything of relevance. More disturbing, 55% of basic clinical information, such as standard medical and surgical treatments for breast cancer, was thought to be inadequate, and 24% of the time these basics were omitted. The authors note that the situation is even worse for Spanish-language Web sites, and conclude that those using the Internet to find medical information "may have a difficult time finding complete and accurate information on a health problem."

But we can't ignore the Internet. It is too powerful and too useful. In the next section, I will discuss some tips on how to use the Internet with a minimum of risk. Following that, I will discuss some specific Web sites that I think are useful and reliable. Be aware, however, that discussing the Internet is like taking aim at a moving target: It may not be in the same place twice.

By all means, use the Internet. But be careful.

BEWARE THE INTERNET

The Internet is full of information, informed opinions, and powerful tools that can help you. It is also chock-full of medical nonsense that can harm you and riddled with scams designed to take your money and rip you off.

Let me say that again: The Internet is chock-full of medical nonsense that can harm you and riddled with scams designed to take your money and rip you off.

As we pointed out in the last section, the problem is that the Internet is completely unregulated. Anyone can put anything they like on the Web, and with today's software they can easily make it look appealing and professional. There is a lot of junk and misinformation out there, placed by those who are well meaning but misinformed. And there are a lot of deliberate lies on the Web, put there by unscrupulous criminals who only want to make a dollar out of your medical misfortune. To make matters worse, it can be difficult or impossible to tell the legitimate Web sites apart from the crooks.

So what can you do? Probably the best defense is to remain skeptical. If a site makes claims that are too good to be true, they are probably false. If a site wants you to buy something, send money, or release your personal information, think twice. If you cannot identify the sponsor of a Web site, move on. And be suspicious of sponsors that are unknown to you or have corporate interests.

The problem of medical misinformation and fraud on the Web has become so rampant that several excellent Web sites have been created just to help you with these problems. A superb site is Quackwatch (www.quackwatch.org). Founded by Dr. Stephen Barrett in 1969, Quackwatch is described as "Your guide to health fraud, quackery, and intelligent decisions." It is an incorporated entity, a member of numerous councils against medical fraud, and a reliable source of information about questionable medical practices. Here you will find myriad articles on everything from colloidal solutions to dubious advertising, along with advice on how to avoid being cheated and how to find a doctor.

Be alert. Be skeptical. There are bad guys out there, waiting to deceive you. Don't let them.

The Internet is a cruel place.

TIPS FOR INTERNET USE

The Internet is vast and our lives are short. Accordingly, my first piece of advice is to limit the number of Web sites you use routinely. Find a few general medical Web sites that you like and use those to find more specialized sites as you require. It is like picking a route to get to work; you would exhaust yourself if you had to find a completely new set of streets every day.

Likewise, limit yourself to a small number of search engines. It takes a while to develop a feel for what kind of information each engine brings and how it is organized. Unless you have a lot of free time, it is more efficient to obtain this experience with just a few of the many available search engines, such as Google, Altavista, or Yahoo. Other so-called metaengines search through many ordinary engines for their results. These include Dogpile, 37, and IxQuick. There are more. And don't forget that many medical Web sites contain specialized search engines that are worth investigating.

Whenever you use a Web site, be aware of who pays for it. I've always been skeptical when a Web site sponsored by an HMO tells me which operations are really medically necessary, or when a pharmaceutical Web site tells me which drugs really work. Web sites with lots of advertising and "buy now" clicks also arouse my suspicions. But you need to set your own level of skepticism. Each Web site should have a page revealing its sponsors, sometimes labeled "About Us." If you can't determine who sponsors your site, I'd give serious consideration to moving on to the next. And there is always a next.

Web sites maintained by patients with specific medical problems are becoming more common. There are those devoted to diabetes, to heart disease, and even to a number of very rare tumors. These sites can be valuable sources of information, provide links to medical centers with special expertise, and offer much-needed personal and emotional support. At the risk of angering some of these very worthy groups, I want to point out that there is no way to evaluate the quality of technical information they offer, nor of the qualifications of their authors. As always, investigate what you learn.

There are also a number of Web sites that will provide you with search results for a one-time or monthly fee. Some of these may be useful to professional librarians or researchers, but I do not believe they will be necessary for you. The existing search engines are quite enough, more than you can completely use in one lifetime.

Some Web sites offer to conduct a search or to perform some calculations just for you. They will ask for some personal information, perhaps height and weight or your name and address. Don't do it. Privacy is a huge issue on the Internet, and rules have not been established. You have little assurance that your personal data won't become public or be used for other purposes without your knowledge. My advice is to stay anonymous.

Be persistent. There is a lot of commercial gleep out there that can hide what you seek. For example: I used Altavista to conduct a search for keratoconus, a malady of the cornea that impairs vision. The first few pages contained hundreds of ads for clinics and physicians offering treatment of keratoconus. I had to use a general medical Web site to discover that the National Keratoconus Foundation exists and has a very useful and informative Web site.

Web sites are being used more and more for interactive information. There are "talk to the doctor" Web sites that allow you to obtain on-line consultations with physicians for a fee. I see a lot of problems with this approach, such as brevity and privacy, so I am not its biggest fan. Finally, many doctors are beginning to use email to communicate with their patients. As many as 10% of physicians use email for this purpose, and about 50% of American doctors have Web sites you can visit. Again, there are problems of confidentiality and reliability, and I cannot help but view a doctor's Web site as a bit of an advertisement, but these uses are growing. Talk with your doctors.

The Internet is a powerful but double-edged tool.

Before We Begin: One More Word

As you read the list of Web sites that follow, you may feel overwhelmed. How can you choose where to begin, which of the many Web sites to explore, and in what order to proceed? How can you possibly sort through a twelve-page list of Web sites to find just the information you need without enduring weeks or even months of meticulous reading?

Have no fear. You are quite capable of using the Internet to your benefit, although you may have to change your attitude about data. Here's what I mean.

The Internet is not a book that you can read from start to finish, being one of the few commodities with no beginning and no end. This may be disturbing to those of you (like me!) who like order and who expect to be able to find structure in everything you do. But facts are facts: The information in the Internet is scattered over so many Web sites in so many ways that it will defy any of your attempts to impose order. It is not a meal that begins with an appetizer, progresses through the main course, and ends with coffee and dessert.

But it is like a picnic. Think of the Internet as a giant picnic table, a smorgasbord full of information for you to devour at your leisure. Some of the plates are large, containing main courses—Web sites containing alphabetized lists of comprehensive articles. Others are small, containing condiments that change the main courses from tasty to superlative—more specialized Web sites with more particular—and perhaps less complete—information. And notice that you don't eat at a picnic by starting with food A and going to food Z. Instead, you take a little of one of the main courses, then a side dish, then some catsup, then a second main dish, and then maybe back to the first main dish. You might even eat dessert before you eat your vegetables, depending on your mood. Eating at a picnic is a feat of organized chaos that we all handle quite effortlessly and with contented pleasure.

And so we should with the Internet. Never mind that there are more than a dozen general Web sites in our list, each of them holding enough information to choke a cyborg. Just start with one, read about your topic for a while, print out the parts you like, and move on. Look at a more specialized site, then another general site, then go back to the first; or dig deeper into the first Web site you found and save the others for tomorrow. You don't have to read A to Z, you only have to sample enough to get what you need. Your own style will guide you, just as it does at a picnic table crammed full of goodies. And while it is no fun to be sick or to have a medical problem, you may find that the process of becoming deeply informed about an important topic is empowering, satisfying, and even enjoyable.

Enjoy the hunt.

SUGGESTED MEDICAL WEB SITES

I'll show you my favorite medical Web sites as long as you understand that what I like today might be really awful tomorrow—or might not even still exist. The problem is that Web sites change with such breakneck speed that the ownership, philosophy, and utility of a site can be radically different every time you log on. For that reason, the sites I recommend will either be government sponsored or run by established, reputable companies that should not change too often or too drastically. Just be aware that nothing lasts forever, especially on today's Internet.

General Medical Web Sites: Government-Sponsored
Let's talk about government-sponsored Web sites first. These turn out to be well-organized sources that not only serve the professional medical community, but are also available free of charge to the public. Most of the time they are pleasantly informative and comfortingly free of commercial influence.

Gateway. Without a doubt, the best government site to begin your search is the Gateway Web site of the National Library of Medicine (NLM) (http://gateway.nlm.nih.gov/gw/Cmd [Note: The "C" in Cmd must be capitalized!]). As its name implies, this site is the entrance to a number of excellent resources run by the NLM. You can search through all of these resources at once, or you can use them individually and bookmark them if you want to return to them without going through the main Gateway site. The information available from Gateway is vast and yet so well organized that all the facts seem to flow to you effortlessly. Its resources include access to medical articles, the top medical and health news items, drug updates, and the latest on research trials.

I like the Gateway site and its links because they are well written and trustworthy. And because its sponsor is the NLM, there is little fear of corporate influence. You don't have to give up your personal information to use this site, and it's free.

Let's look at each of the individual sites included in the Gateway menu.

PubMed. My favorite Web site on the Gateway list is PubMed (www.ncbi.nlm.nih.gov/entrez/query.fcgi). This is the NLM site most used to find medical articles, allowing you to search the vast holdings of MEDLINE as well as a collection of nonmedical scientific articles. Since MEDLINE contains more than 12 million articles from 4,500 journals and is updated regularly, PubMed is one of the most popular and essential Internet tools used by all healthcare professionals. Needless to say, it should be high on your list of sources, too. It is easy to use and yet has advanced features if you want to be fancy. It also provides you with a summary of the articles (the Abstract) in most cases, so that you can get the gist of the information without having to find the entire article. This is a tremendous benefit that lets you cover a lot of ground very quickly. I will include some instructions for use in the next section. Bookmark this indispensable site.

MEDLINEplus. Another site on the Gateway list and possibly the most important Web site in this list is MEDLINEplus (www.medlineplus.gov). This well-organized site contains loads of useful information concerning a wide variety of medical topics and is written for the general public. The articles are clear, informative, and worthwhile. MEDLINEplus includes:

+ A collection of short medical articles, arranged alphabetically and equipped with a search engine. You will find something about everything here.

✦ A collection of articles about medications, also arranged alphabetically. Here you can find what you need to know about the drugs you are taking.

✦ A medical encyclopedia, full of medical illustrations and reference information.

✦ A handy medical dictionary (bookmark this for quick access).

✦ A current events section, summarizing the top medical news stories from the past thirty days.

✦ An exhaustive list of links to other Web sites that help you find medical specialists in every conceivable category.

There is a lot of useful information on MEDLINEplus; it's worth checking out.

Clinical Trials. This third member of the Gateway family lets you search for clinical research studies, something you might want to do if you are interested in experimental treatment and new drugs. There is a nice explanation of clinical trials and how to approach participation, and you can browse the site or search by disease or phrase. Like the other Gateway sites, it is both huge and well organized.

Clinical Alert. This Gateway component lists the findings of NIH-funded research thought to be of public interest. It is another good way to keep up to date on topics of interest to you.

Other Gateway sites include ToxNet (a compendium of information about poisons and toxins), HSTAT (a technical but fascinating searchable database of evaluations of various medical treatments), and LocatorPlus (a directory of NLM holdings, complete but only useful if you can visit the National Library of Medicine). All are government sponsored, all are excellent, and all are worth your time, whether you are reading broadly or just need that one bit of special information.

Finally, Gateway has a nice way to obtain copies of the articles you find, especially useful if you cannot easily visit a medical library. This is the Lonesome Doc service (click "Ordering Info"), a site that shows you how to order your copies from selected medical libraries for a small fee. You must register to use this service.

Let's leave Gateway, and look at some other major medical Web sites maintained by the government.

NLM. In addition to maintaining the Gateway site, the National Library of Medicine has its own Web site (www.nlm.nih.gov) full of useful information. There is admittedly some overlap with Gateway, but there are additional features here that Gateway does not have. DIRLINE is a directory of hospitals and health organizations to get you started. NIHSenior Health is a section devoted to health information for older adults, containing some hard-to-find links specifically useful to the senior crowd. NLM also gives you a plethora of links to such diverse topics as AIDS, cancer, public health, space medicine, and arctic medicine.

NIH. At the risk of being redundant, the NIH site (www.nih.gov) is worth knowing about. It can lead you to more explanations of all sorts of medical topics, available clinical studies, drug information, and other medical links. There is some overlap with Gateway and NLM.

HealthFinder. This is a wonderful Web site (www.healthfinder.gov) true to its name; it is designed to help you find reliable medical Web sites, medical agencies and organizations, and physicians. Its extensive holdings are well organized and maintained by the U.S. Department of Health and Human Services. You will find easy access to over 1,800 medical governmental agencies, nonprofit organizations, and universities, as well as explanations of medical topics arranged alphabetically. There are specialty sections addressing specific medical issues for men, women, and children, and a section telling you how and where to find reliable physicians. It also has a handy list of links to other medical sites and organizations. Don't skip this one; it will help you find sites you might otherwise overlook.

FDA. Need some information about new or old drugs? How about experimental or established medical devices? Then this is the Web site (www.fda.gov) for you, full of information for the patient-consumer from the government, unbiased by commercial concerns. You can search its well-organized contents or browse an alphabetical list, and there is even a phone number for specific questions. The list of drugs and devices covered is exhaustive, and the topics include everything from buying medicine online to LASIK surgery. Also provided is access to the official FDA magazine (*FDA Consumer*), an intriguing resource even if it is a bit difficult to use.

General Medical Web Sites: Non–Government-Sponsored

Let's now discuss some nongovernmental medical Web sites. Here we can't afford to ignore the question of who pays for the sites and who maintains them, and not all Web sites are equally credible. The choices I made are based on my personal preferences and cannot be all-inclusive, since there are literally thousands of excellent medical Web sites devoted to every conceivable medical topic. You will notice that I stay away from sites run by insurance companies, sites constructed with the goal of selling you something, and sites with a lot of commercials and pop-up windows; it's hard enough to find good medical information without the distraction of a sales pitch. To that end, I will tell you who maintains the Web site whenever I can. I will also avoid sites that seem to be all interpretation and no data; you never know who is doing the interpreting and what their agenda might be.

Let's start with Web sites that are not specialized. These will give you general information about a wide variety of medical topics and provide you with links to others. These are great places to begin.

HealthWeb. Like Healthfinder (see above), HealthWeb is another marvelous Web site (www.healthweb.org) designed to help you find medical information and agencies. It is maintained by a collaboration between the health science libraries of the Greater MidWest Region, the National Network of Libraries of Medicine, and the Committee for Institutional Cooperation, and is supported by the National Library of Medicine. It contains many great links to medical topics and articles, arranged alphabetically. I think this is one of the best; it will quickly propel you to lots of reputable, reliable, and relevant medical Web sites.

HardinMD. This Web site (www.lib.uiowa.edu/hardin/md) is a superb collection of links to important medical Web sites, arranged alphabetically by disease. It is maintained by the Hardin Library for the Health Sciences at the University of Iowa, and seems to be free of troublesome commercial influences. You can use the many links here to begin your search. It has a hard-to-find list of medical journals that offer their articles for free.

UTSouthwestern. Another Web site chock-full of useful links is maintained by the University of Texas Southwestern Medical Center (www2.utsouthwestern.edu). The list is a bit hard to find (look under

Resources, then Library, then More Subjects), but this alphabetized treasure-trove is well worth the trouble.

Mayo Clinic. The Mayo Clinic Web site (www.mayohealth.org) contains many nice articles about a variety of medical topics. Lists of Mayo Clinic physicians are sprinkled throughout and may be useful if you are thinking of being seen there.

YaleHealth. Want to know the difference between an MRI and a CBC? Look here. This site (www.yalenewhavenhealth.org) not only gives you information about medical conditions and drugs, but also sports a rarely found section about medical tests. This university-maintained medical Web site is worth knowing about.

WebMDHealth. This commercial Web site (www.webmd.com) is supported by a number of medical business entities and contains a vast amount of well-written medical information. You will find articles on specific medical topics and guides to clinical trials and wellness. There is an opportunity to become a WebMD member, although, as always, make sure you completely understand the terms before sharing any personal information.

Virtual Hospital. This gem of a Web site (www.vh.org) is maintained by the University of Iowa and provides lots of outstanding articles about medical topics. What makes this site unique are some sections not easily found elsewhere. For example, not only is there a useful section devoted to pediatrics, but also a section meant to be read by children explaining a host of medical conditions and their treatment in gentle ways kids will understand. Click on *Virtual Children's Hospital* at the top of the Web page, then find the *For Kids* section. Their wonderful atlas of human anatomy beautifully illustrates all the nooks and crannies of the human body.

Family Doctor. Another gem (there are so many!), maintained by the American Academy of Family Physicians and devoted to providing you with reliable information on general medical topics: No concern is too big or too small for this Web site (www.familydoctor.org). True to its name, its extensive holdings include medical problems of children as well as a lot of health issues you may have wondered about but never gotten around to asking your doctor. Check those out here.

Merck Manual. The various editions of this thick, encyclopedic manual have been a standard reference for diseases and their treatment for more than 100 years. Limited portions of the new 2003 second edition of the *Merck Manual of Diagnosis and Therapy* are now available on the Web site (www.merck.com) maintained by Merck & Company. The 1999 edition of the book is also available in its entirety, complete with a search engine, on the same site. Be aware that the information in this latter edition is a few years old, but it is a good starting point for your reading and you can find it whenever you want for free. Keep this site in mind.

Web Sites for Medical Reference

Here are a few Web sites providing you with background material and reference information that may be helpful during your medical quest.

Medical Dictionary. I mentioned this earlier, but don't forget the medical dictionary available on MEDLINEplus (www.medlineplus. gov).

Anatomy. Bartleby maintains a Web site (www.bartleby.com) that offers the full and complete 1918 edition of *Gray's Anatomy*. Admittedly, this edition of *the* classic and comprehensive anatomy book is a bit dated, but the human body has not changed that much in 100 years. This site might be worth a look for those quick questions about anatomy.

Books. The government-maintained Web site of the National Center for Biotechnology Information (www.ncbi.nlm.nih.gov) keeps a long list of medical books available for your reading free of charge. Most are a bit off our track, but a few (such as *Cancer Medicine* and *Genes and Disease)* might be relevant to your needs.

Practice Guidelines. The University of California at San Francisco maintains this Web site (http://medicine.ucsf.edu/resources/guide lines/), making you privy to the guidelines recommended to doctors for the treatment of a host of medical conditions. The contents of this site are unique—they will give you a flavor of the strategy your doctor may use to help you with your medical problem. Just remember that guidelines are only suggested recommendations and may not apply verbatim to every case.

Guideline Database. The National Guidelines Clearing House (www.guideline.gov) is a government-maintained searchable database containing guidelines for treatment of a wide variety of medical problems. It is a bit difficult to use but can yield some fascinating data.

Web Sites for Specific Conditions

There are many, many Web sites for specific diseases such as diabetes, arthritis, or lung disease. Those maintained by government or professional organizations—the American Medical Association, for example—are usually worth checking out, but are too numerous to list here. I've listed some of these to give you an idea of what is available; links to others can be found in the general Web sites we discussed earlier.

American Heart Association. This is the official site of the American Heart Association (www.americanheart.org) and contains a ton of terrific information about heart attacks and heart disease. There are sections showing you how to assess your risk of having a heart attack and explanations on how to achieve a heart-healthy lifestyle. Quite a helpful Web site for any type of heart disease.

American Stroke Association. This is the official site of the American Stroke Association (www.strokeassociation.org), similar in style and organization to that of the American Heart Association. This is a must-look for anyone concerned about stroke.

American Diabetes Association. The official site of the American Diabetes Association (http://diabetes.org) is where you look for the most up-to-date information about diabetes and its treatment.

National Institute of Diabetes and Digestive and Kidney Diseases. The government-maintained Web site for the NIDDK (www.niddk.nih.gov/) is another superlative resource for those concerned with diabetes. Lots of information about diabetes and an essential section about the natural history of this all-too-common disease.

National Cancer Institute. This site (www.cancer.gov) is a rich source of information about cancer and its treatment. You can find explanations of hundreds of types of cancer, links to and lists of clinical trials and research programs, and an understandable (really!) section about the medical statistics that are so important to interpreting cancer research. If you are thinking about enrolling in a research protocol, there is also a very thoughtful section about how to find these research programs and how to choose the one that's right for you. It includes a frank discussion of the financial aspects of this decision.

The Susan G. Komen Breast Cancer Foundation. This organization has long been an inspiring light for those concerned with breast cancer, and their Web site (www.komen.org) shines even farther. Check this out for all aspects of breast cancer and its treatment.

AIDSinfo. Here you can find huge amounts of information and a long list of links addressing every aspect of AIDS and its treatment. This government-maintained site (www.aidsinfo.nih.gov) is a great resource for anyone needing information about this devastating illness.

National Institute of Mental Health. The general medical Web sites do not always include an in-depth coverage of psychiatric problems, so it is good to know about the Web site of the National Institute of Mental Health (www.nimh.nih.gov). Here you will find reliable information and a list of compassionate resources to help with the entire spectrum of psychiatric and psychological illness.

Office of Rare Diseases. Didn't find what you needed in the Web sites so far? It's possible that your medical problem is so rare that it is not covered by the usual sources. If so, look at this excellent Web site maintained by the government and devoted to rare diseases (http://rarediseases.info.nih.gov/). In addition to giving you lots of useful information and providing you with links to specialized and hard-to-find Web sites, it offers a list of links to research trials, and tells you how to find the support groups that can be so important to those with rare medical problems. Keep this one in mind if you are having trouble finding good information about your medical needs.

Web Sites for Specific Interests

There are also scads of Web sites devoted to specific populations or concerns. Although I advise consulting a general medical Web site first, some of these specialty Web sites are magnificent and should not be ignored. Here are a few.

4Woman. This Web site (www.4woman.gov) is devoted to women's medical issues. Maintained by the U.S. Department of Health and Human Services, it offers a searchable list of articles on medical topics about women's health—everything from breast cancer to diabetes to hormone replacement therapy. It sponsors a toll-free call center for specific questions, and is an essential resource for information about women's health.

KidsHealth. Medicine for children is its own specialty, and this huge Web site (www.kidshealth.org) is devoted to pediatric issues. It is well organized and searchable, and contains hundreds of articles about medical issues of babies and children that you may not find on the more general medical Web sites. It is maintained by the Nemours Foundation and should be on your list if you are making medical decisions for children. (Don't forget about the *Virtual Hospital* and *Family Doctor* Web sites for information about the medical problems of children.)

National Center for Complementary and Alternative Medicine. There is no other aspect within medicine that invites more abuse, more fraud, and more outright lying than alternative medicine. It is all too easy to find Web sites that are either well meaning but ill-informed, or well informed but deliberately misleading. But this reliable site (http://nccam.nih.gov), maintained by the National Center for Complementary and Alternative Medicine, focuses fairly and impartially on these important topics. Here you will find treatments that you may never have heard of, as well as informed discussions of their pros and cons.

CDC. The Centers for Disease Control and Prevention maintains an excellent Web site (www.cdc.gov) on the topics of infection and contagious diseases. You can find current information about travel risks and recommendations, public health issues, and terrorism in addition to the latest efforts to control infectious disease of all types.

HOW TO SEARCH THE WEB FOR MEDICAL WEB SITES

As I commented earlier, there is a lot of junk on the Internet, and finding a good Web site will require some dedicated and careful searching. One approach is to use some of the Web sites listed in the last section that contain links to other Web sites with medical information. These include Healthfinder, Healthweb, HardinMD, and UTSouthwestern.

These sites are responsibly maintained and strive to include links to only the most reputable Web sites. Remember that it makes sense to use just a few familiar sites rather than taking the trouble of finding new ones each time.

But on occasion you will want more specific information, or maybe you just want to see what else is out there. Then you will use one of the Web search engines we have mentioned, such as Google or Altavista, to do your search. It is best to start with a specific search topic. A search for "cancer," for example, will pull up so many Web sites it would take you years to see them all. Even a more specific search such as "breast cancer" or "cancer drugs" will be overwhelming.

One way around this is to ignore most of the search results, using only the first few Web pages appearing in your search. This will often direct you to reputable sites, but beware: the order in which Web sites appear in a search is not a matter of chance. Organizations pay top dollar to be listed first, so that the most useful sites to you might be buried down around page 20. You may also find that the first few pages are often filled with advertisements for medical products or services that are irrelevant to your medical decisions.

Another strategy is to narrow your search topic by using search words that are specialized, such as "arrhythmia" or "melanoma." The result should be a shorter, more focused list of Web sites. Or you can combine search topics. Some search engines allow you to do this by typing a "+" between two topics. Web sites appearing in a search for "breast cancer + surgery," for example, must have references to both breast cancer and surgery. The resulting list is smaller than for "breast cancer" or "surgery" alone.

You must also decide if a particular Web site is worth your time. Some are filled with commercials or wild claims, and are easy to spot. Others are advertisements for medications or hospitals, and are rarely helpful. Be sure to find out who sponsors and pays for the site, and how often it is updated.

We cannot escape the fact that there is a lot of information on the Web, no matter how lean and efficient our searches become. Sifting through these sites takes time and energy. But no one said that the search for good medical information wouldn't take legwork. The best things in life, and the best searches, take time.

Good searches are not easy.

How to Look at a Medical Web Site

Now that you've found a promising medical Web site, how do you use it?

The good news is that many medical Web sites are intricate works of art, miraculously weaving vital medical facts within a gorgeous presentation that would make Michelangelo weep. The bad news is that even Michelangelo would get confused; all this weaving of information can be overwhelming, so much so that it is hard to know where to start, what to read, or how to get there. There seem to be so many tabs to click, so many choices—how do you decide which medical headlines to read, or which Web site features to explore first? How can you avoid overlooking something that might be lifesaving? Is it desirable or even possible to start at the beginning and read everything?

Well, most medical Web sites are so vast that you cannot read every bit of information they offer. Instead, I recommend that you think of a medical Web site the way you think of something you use without much thought all the time: the grocery store. A modern grocery store is also a work of art, weaving thousands of food items together within gorgeous presentation that would at least make Michelangelo hungry. We find our way around these intricate markets with ease (although finding the occasional odd bottle of hot sauce can be frustrating), largely because of their organization into aisles of similar foods. And we almost never find potatoes by starting at one corner of the grocery and laboriously examining each item until we find the spud section; we would die of starvation first.

A medical Web site can be mastered just as easily as you master the grocery store. Each feature—the library of articles, or the medical dictionary, or the anatomy atlas—is like a grocery aisle containing similar items. Go down one aisle to find what you need, then go down another if you can't find just the right thing, then return to the first if a different idea strikes you. It is just like shopping for dinner. Only easier, because most Web sites have nifty tools to help find your way. For example, the name of a section will change color once you visit it, so you can tell where you have been. And many Web sites contain a map (click on *site map*) which lays out its entire plan so you can get your bearings. Finally, most Web sites allow you to search for specific terms like "arthritis" or "cancer"; it is like asking the grocery clerk to point you to the potatoes.

Just as we don't eat our meals right off the grocery shelf—most of us use a shopping cart—so we cannot expect to digest all the medical information we find on a Web site as we explore its contents. Instead of a cart, you have several options. You can take notes as you go, or you can save the text for your own use later (if the Web site allows this, of course). And you can use your browser to bookmark specific pages of interest. But often the easiest way is to print the text of interest (again, if the Web site allows you to do so). That way you can read the information later, at your leisure, several times if needed.

So don't be afraid of medical Web sites, since they are usually interesting and often exciting. Browse and peruse and stroll through them as you would a grocery store; all the medical information you need is waiting for you on the shelf.

The medical Web site is an information grocery store.

HOW TO USE PUBMED

I want to focus on PubMed because it is a reliable search engine for MEDLINE, used by almost every doctor in the world to access medical literature. PubMed has as many sophisticated features as you could ever desire, but is also easy and intuitive to use. It contains an excellent Help section, complete with examples and tutorials. Here I will give just a few tips.

Your search results will be more helpful if you use specific topics. A search for "cancer" will bring forth too many articles to read in any one lifetime. You can also search for a particular author or a particular medical journal, or even a medical phrase such as "heart disease in children."

PubMed allows you to combine search items by simply listing the different topics. For example, "breast cancer surgery complications" will find articles about all three of these topics. You can also type the word "AND" between the topics to restrict attention to articles that address all of them. Typing "heart AND exercise" will list articles focusing on both the heart and exercise. Most of the time this will result in a more manageable list of articles that are focused to your needs. A nice trick is to include the word "review" in your search, making it more likely to find articles written to review the field. Remember, review articles are useful because they often contain a balanced discussion about different options and opinions. A search under "heart failure AND drugs AND review" might pull forth review articles on medications used for heart failure. PubMed allows you to be fancy with "OR" and "NOT" operators, too. Read about them in the Help section.

Be creative. Try to think of different combinations of topics, and don't be afraid to conduct many searches. PubMed is quick, and even ten or twenty searches won't take long. Articles you have already viewed are highlighted on your subsequent searches, a convenience keeping you from duplicating your work.

Your search results are listed by relevance, but they can also be listed in chronological order with the most recent articles first (click on "Sort," then choose "Pub Date," then click on "Display"). By clicking on the title, you can read the abstract, if it is available, and choose whether to print it. Remember that it is not necessary to understand all of an abstract in order to obtain useful information. A quick scan of the abstract will help you determine if you want a copy of the article for yourself.

PubMed will display twenty items at a time unless you specify otherwise. I find it convenient to display more, preferring one long download rather than many shorter ones. Having seen the entire list, you can mark those you want to save on the PubMed clipboard and print them all later at your convenience.

Each listing of an article is accompanied by a "related articles" option. Clicking here will produce a list of articles with the same focus as the chosen one, helping you to find lots of additional information on a particular topic.

Many other features of PubMed are nicely described in its Tutorial and Help sections. You can limit your searches to human studies, save and combine different searches, and keep a history of your own efforts. Although many physicians (myself included) get along quite well with only the simple features of PubMed, you can be as elaborate as you like.

Once you have chosen your articles, you can look them up at the local medical library or use the services provided by PubMed to obtain your copy. Lonesome Doc, for example, allows you to obtain copies of articles by mail, fax, or email for a fee. You must first register with a medical library of your choice. These are convenient services, but a visit to your local medical library may be easier and quicker.

Try PubMed; you'll like it.

Final Words

Finding good information on the Internet is an art that no one ever completely masters. Do not despair if the going is slow. Persistence and legwork will pay off with good Web sites and reliable information.

And don't despair if it seems that you have found a lot of data but you really don't know how to evaluate it or what it means. We will pay great attention to these problems in later chapters.

FRIENDS AND FAMILY

Let's leave behind the electronic sources for a moment, and consider some of our most treasured sources of information and opinion: friends and family.

Individuals

Pat D. is sitting on a wooden bench in the locker room in his underwear, carefully massaging his right knee after a long workout. He exercises in this gym religiously, favoring a combination of stair stepper aerobics and weight lifting. Unfortunately, the pain in his knee has been increasing, limiting his exercise more and more. After consulting with several orthopedic surgeons and roaming the Internet for hours, he has scheduled himself for a knee surgery tomorrow morning. Today is his last workout for a while, and only the nagging pain in his knee is preventing him from savoring it.

A friend passes by the bench on the way from the showers. "What's the deal with your knee?" Pat explains about the pain and how he hopes the surgery will restore his ability to exercise. But his friend stops and frowns, asking, "Have you tried that new cartilage pill? My elbow hurt for a long time, and it worked for me." He pauses. "You ought to try it."

Pat keeps rubbing his knee, and replies thoughtfully, "Really? Maybe I ought to check that out." And the next day he postpones his surgery so that he can investigate the use of cartilage.

Lynn S. is a 34-year-old woman who is in my office to discuss possible surgery. She has brought her friend Jackie for moral support. After hearing the details and risks, Lynn decides to have the surgery and wants to schedule a date. Jackie reminds her to pick a day during a certain astrological phase, and Lynn is grateful for her reminder.

A truly powerful source of information can be found from the opinions that come from our friends and family. Even in the age of the Internet and of technical medicine, we look to the people in our lives for truthful information and direction. We have always been and always will be social animals.

And no wonder. Our friends and family are the only people in the world with our best interests at heart. Husbands and wives look after each other when they are ill and support each other through difficult decisions. Parents guard their children from medical harm, and children make medical decisions for their aging parents. Friends are genuine in their wish to provide helpful advice and concern. Even casual acquaintances can be selflessly informative and protective. Pat, for example, learned from a friend about a new medication that might help his knee without surgery. Lynn was reminded by her friend to make arrangements in accord with her philosophy of life.

But there are problems with the medical information we receive from friends and family, just as there are problems from any source. First is the fact that no one knows you as well as you do. The most well-meaning friends and the closest of family members still cannot know all of your wishes, needs, and expectations. And it is you, not they, who will live with the consequences of your medical decisions. Advice from others can therefore never be perfect.

Another problem is that your friends and family often assume that their likes and dislikes are the same as yours. Psychologists have noted that most people assume that their own opinions are more common than they really are. They call this the *false consensus effect*. An example is the teenager who assumes that everyone likes loud music, or the political liberal who cannot really believe that anyone could be conservative. If our friends or family harbor mistaken assumptions about our beliefs and needs, their most heartfelt advice may well miss the mark.

It is also true that information received from our well-intentioned friends and family may be incorrect. The information we hear in our casual conversation is of course not scrutinized for scientific rigor, and could be filled with fallacy and exaggeration. It may be something they simply overheard or believe for unclear reasons. Pat found this out when he discovered later that the evidence for the success of those cartilage pills was really quite shaky. And even if your friends have splendid intentions, your medical results might not be the same as theirs. To make matters worse, advice from friends or family is frequently delivered with a sense of absolute authority, even if the advice itself is poor.

But the fact remains that the people who love you and nurture you in this world are your friends and family. They are the people with your interests in mind, and they are indeed a powerful source of information and support.

Listen to your friends and family, but listen with a grain of salt.

GROUPS

Walter W. is a 67-year-old man with a devastating hand tremor, waiting with his extended family in my office. With him is his wife, brother, two sons and their wives, his daughter and her husband, and a small grandson who is occasionally taken into the hallway to play. Walter and his wife are seated in the small examining room, and there is standing room only for the others. They listen carefully as I explain the surgery for tremor, and they are even more attentive when I review the risks. Each of them has some questions, which are answered one by one. At the end of this discussion, it is Walter's wife's turn to speak. She is smaller than he is, with neatly trimmed white hair and a quick manner that contrasts with Walter's deliberate and slow ways. She turns to him and asks, "Walter, do you want to have this surgery?" Then she looks over at me, smiling, and says "It's really his decision. I can't decide for him."

After a pause, Walter tells his family that he is tired of living with his tremor, and that he wants to have the surgery. They nod in silent agreement. Some of them catch my eye as if to reinforce their approval. I then ask him, "Which side would you like us to do? If we operate on the left side of your brain, we will treat the tremor in your right hand." Walter thinks for a moment, and says, "My left hand bothers me more. Let's do that one."

There was a long silence in the room, as the family hesitantly looked at one another. His daughter finally spoke up, saying, "But, Daddy, the tremor is really worse in your right hand." His wife pitched in, "Walter, what are you saying? You can't even hold a fork with your right hand. Why would you want them to fix your left hand?" One of his sons frowned to himself, as if he disagreed with the others, but kept silent. Then Walter pleaded, "But I can't use my left hand in my shop."

I assured the family that I would be happy to operate on either side, then excused myself while they continued their discussion. When I returned, they informed me that he wanted his right hand treated. But Walter did not look happy, and neither did some other members of his family. I decided to discuss the issue with him again at a later time when he and I could talk alone.

Special problems arise when decisions are made by groups. Many people feel reluctant to share their true opinions when they are together with you and others, since they are afraid of looking silly or hurting your feelings. You will therefore not receive the honest feedback that could be helpful. Other people will "loaf" in a group, seeming to agree with the consensus opinion and allowing one particular aggressive person to dominate. And neither groups nor individuals can always know the right decision for you. Walter's wife was right to say that she could not decide for him.

Group decisions can be unpredictable and do not always reflect the opinions of their individual members. For example, social psychologists have shown that the decisions arising from groups are often more risky than those chosen by the individual member. In one study, a group of people was willing to accept more risks of an open heart surgery for a hypothetical patient than they would as individuals. This would be of clear importance to you if the group in question was your family, discussing the amount of risk that you should take.

Another example of poor group decisions arises from what Irving Janus has termed *groupthink*, a problem occurring when some members of a group are so confident of their decisions that the other members remain silent. The most famous example of poor decisions due to groupthink is the series of choices made in the Bay of Pigs incident in the 1960s, decisions that very nearly led to a nuclear war. An interesting solution to the problem of groupthink has been creatively addressed by some Japanese organizations, which require their junior members to speak first at a meeting so that they are not influenced by the opinions of their seniors.

Peer pressure is another force operating in groups that may stifle honest opinion. This was dramatically demonstrated in the now classic experiments of Solomon Asch, in which small groups of people were asked to compare the lengths of two lines drawn on a piece of paper. All but one in the group were in fact conspirators with Asch, and were instructed to deliberately voice the wrong answer. For example, the conspirators would be instructed to say that the longer line was in fact the shorter of the two. Amazingly, the one person being tested would often agree with the group of conspirators, calling the long line short despite obvious evidence to the contrary.

Each of us benefits from the advice and support of the groups around us. But group decisions are not necessarily the wisest or best for us as individuals. In the next section, we will discuss some ways around these problems.

Two heads aren't always better than one.

How to Benefit from Friends and Family

Several strategies can lessen the problems of group decisions and help you benefit from the insights and strong resources inherent in friends and family.

Check it out yourself. As for any source of information, check it out for yourself. Your well-meaning friend or cousin might tell you about new treatments, but it is up to you to investigate them and verify that they are valid for you. Your friends and family can be invaluable eyes and ears, as long as you maintain a healthy skepticism.

Seek advice but make your own decisions. Go ahead and ask for advise from friends and family, but realize that you have to make your own decisions. Ask how they have solved their own medical problems, keeping in mind that their solutions may not be right for you. It is your life and your body, even if it is true that you can benefit from the advice and experience of others.

Ask your close friends or family to play devil's advocate. Ask them to gently challenge your opinions and encourage you to justify your plans. Once your friends or family see that you are open to all ideas, they may be encouraged to offer their honest opinions.

Talk with each member of your group individually. Speaking with friends and family one-on-one will help avoid peer pressure and encourage expression of honest opinion. And hearing the private thoughts of the more shy members may help eliminate groupthink. Be especially careful to obtain opinions from the quiet members of the group—they will often harbor the most interesting and provocative thoughts.

Give special consideration to friends and family who are in the medical profession. Insiders can guide you to the best doctors and steer you away from bad decisions. Be aware that they may not have expertise in your particular problem, and that they may feel uncomfortable being completely frank and honest. But they should be able to offer you some insights difficult to obtain elsewhere.

Groups require work.

YOUR DOCTORS

If you haven't been able to guess my opinion about doctors yet, I'll state it clearly here: Your doctors are some of the most important sources of information around. Use them to gather data, use them to seek perspective, and use them to test your ideas and plans. Use more than one doctor, as one person cannot possibly know every fact and viewpoint. And use them to help evaluate your other sources of information. They do their jobs day in and day out, and they have wisdom to share.

In fact, doctors play such an important part in our medical decisions that Part III of this book is dedicated solely to their use.

Don't forget the doctor.

A SUGGESTED STRATEGY FOR FINDING MEDICAL INFORMATION

There are as many ways to weave the use of these sources together as there are to build a house, and everyone will develop their own strategy. Here is just one example.

The basic strategy I prefer is to bounce back and forth among sources. Don't limit yourself to reading the medical textbooks just once; return to them several times, for different types of information. Use the Internet frequently, and arrange to have several conversations with your doctors.

For example, you might begin with the Internet to gain some basic information. MEDLINEplus might be a good place to start, using its comprehensive collection of articles on medical topics. A preliminary search in Gateway or PubMed (using the "AND review" trick) might also turn up some information. The next step would be to find your topic in a medical textbook. Remember that you can find these at your local medical school or hospital library. You may wish to copy parts of these chapters for more leisurely reading.

Questions will arise at this point in your search. How good is surgery, really? What other types of medications are available? And then it's time for a discussion with your doctor.

It may also be time for a more focused search with PubMed. Now that you have identified some specific questions (and also identified your options and risks, as advised in Steps 1 and 6), more specialized articles might be helpful. Once you find the articles on the Internet, you can look them up in your library or order them through a service such as Lonesome Doc.

In the meantime, talk with your friends and family. They may have some new ideas or may have heard of some new medical information. Don't neglect these important informal sources of information.

Then go back to the textbooks to learn some general background. Learn about how the heart works if you have congestive failure, or learn about ARDS (a serious lung problem) if your loved one has been severely injured. A small amount of effort here will really pay off.

Then go back to your doctors again, bringing them the information you have uncovered and discussing your options once more.

You get the idea. Using medical sources is not a step-wise task of books first, then articles, then doctors. You must bounce back and forth among the sources as your need for information changes and as you learn more about the field. The more complex and serious your medical problems, the more bouncing around you must do. This will come quite naturally; don't be afraid to let it happen.

Bounce around.

EIGHT

Step 4: Interpretation of Numbers

THERE ARE TWO distinct tasks wrapped up in the interpretation of data. The first is to cultivate a certain amount of healthy skepticism, because it would be foolish to believe that all facts were equally reliable, or that every interpretation is equally valid. The second task we must face is to master a small amount of mathematical analysis. Data, after all, are made of numbers, and so we will need some statistical tools. Like many topics with mathematical flavor, this task could be dry and boring; we'll try to keep it short and interesting.

—BUILDING SKEPTICISM—

It is difficult to be skeptical of everything. Sure, it is easy enough to dig in your heels and believe nothing you read or hear, but then we would never learn anything. Instead, we need to cultivate our skills at being selective, believing what seems true but able to uncover hidden assumptions that might alter our interpretations. This skill comes more easily to some than others, but is needed by all to make sense of the numerical data thrown at us by modern medical writing.

Trust No One, Believe Nothing

One of the most important principles of medicine I ever learned was taught to me when I worked in a public hospital long ago: "Trust no one, believe nothing." The facility was an aging hospital, lacking proper funds, overstretched to serve its thousands of patients. Years of mismanagement and indifference had taken their toll, playing havoc with the quality of medical care. The hundreds of daily reports of laboratory tests were not stored on a computer; instead, a mass of printed reports was sent unfiled to the ward, crumpled in random order in cardboard boxes, making it inevitable that critical results would go unnoticed. Medications reported as taken by the patients were often not given at all, and measurements of blood pressure and pulse were sometimes fabricated for patients who had in fact died hours before. I can even remember finding living insects swimming in bottles of IV fluid dripping into our patients. Corners were routinely cut in the rush to care for too many people with too little money. Hence it was easy for those of us charged with the bottom line of patient care to become more than a little paranoid and cynical.

We had a motto, beyond the cynicism, in which lived a terrific lesson that undoubtedly saved innumerable lives: *Trust no one, believe nothing.* Verify and confirm every scrap of information for yourself. In the complex, unregulated chaos of that hospital so many years ago, this ensured that physicians would receive accurate information and that important medical interventions would in fact be carried out.

Fortunately, these horror stories are things of the past. But now we have new horror stories, arising from a medical world based on a mass of data, facts, and information that has exploded beyond our capacity to grasp it as a whole. And the same indifference and deceit that were present in those hospitals of long ago can still be found, inflamed anew by commercial greed. Medical opinions based on nothing at best and commercial interests at worst are routinely broadcast in newspapers and on television; whole books of medical nonsense fill the shelves at bookstores; and medical information on the Internet frequently consists of nothing more than thinly disguised advertising. Even if you disagree with my opinion of what is nonsense and what isn't, it is hard to deny that much of the medical information out there is as commercially motivated as a used-car lot. And for me, that means that much of what we are told is unreliable, untrustworthy, and downright scary.

So, I recommend that you be as paranoid and cynical about interpreting medical information as you can bring yourself to be. It may help to pretend that you are deciding about an investment, and that your decision involves money. Don't trust your neighbor or family to have up-to-date, accurate medical facts; don't trust medical books to be unbiased; give a hard eye to medical articles, scientific or otherwise; and above all, think twice about information you receive on the Internet. You wouldn't buy a car or house with any less attitude, and you shouldn't choose your medical care any less stringently. Trust no one, believe nothing.

Check for yourself.

. . . But You Must Trust Your Sources

Although it's good to be hard-nosed, it is sometimes better to be pragmatic. Yes, we need to be skeptical about the medical information we receive, and yes, there is a lot of medical trash and deception out there. But you can drive yourself to unhappiness if all you feel is paranoia and cynicism. At some point, we have to accept what we have.

Once you have done your best to gain good medical information, it is time to relax and use that information in your search for good decisions. The information may be imperfect, as when the efficacy of a particular operation can only be estimated broadly between 50 and 70%. But it does little good to keep on ranting and raving at your information sources when you have done your best and there is no better information available. At this point, it is time to accept the imperfections of the information and use the rest of the tools we are presenting in this book to arrive at decisions that are right for you.

Too much skepticism is as bad as too little.

Go Beyond Words

Let's say you've broken your leg, and your doctor is explaining the different types of treatment. You can choose to have an operation called an FPF (femur-preserving fusion), which works most of the time but has a long recovery. Or you can choose a sarcogenic transplant, which takes less time but doesn't work quite as often. Or you can decide against surgery, and let your leg heal in a Holcomb semirigid brace.

Without reading any further until you decide (no peeking!), which of these options would you choose?

If you chose any of these options, you will be interested to learn that none of them really exists. As far as I know, there is no such thing as an FPF, a sarcogenic transplant, or a Holcomb semirigid brace. They are all completely made up, and yet you were willing to choose one as your treatment.

And you are not alone. Many people are willing to make decisions based on words alone. In a startling study by psychologist Eugene Hartley in 1946, subjects were asked to rate groups of Danireans, Pireneans, and Wallonians on a scale of social distance. They found that 80% of the subjects were able to do so. The only problem was that there is no such thing as Danireans, Pireneans, or Wallonians. They don't exist, any more than sarcogenic transplants or Holcomb semirigid braces do.

Unless you are a professional with expertise in your own illness, the medications and treatments you find will be unfamiliar to you. Before making any decisions, learn what these terms mean, what the treatments in fact are, and something about how they work and their complications. Don't guess at the risks; you'll be wrong most of the time. All of this may sound obvious, but you don't want to end up in a Holcomb semirigid brace. Especially since it doesn't exist.

Make sure you know what you're talking about.

It's All in How You Say It

You are in the doctor's office, and he is telling you about a new medicine that is available to treat the irregularities in your heart rhythm. "Unfortunately," he says, "about ten percent of the people who take this drug die anyway." You thank him quietly without really meaning it, and leave his office to ponder your choices.

Later that week, you are in a second doctor's office to hear another opinion about this same new drug. This doctor says, "Great news! More than ninety percent of people with your condition who take this medication go on to live full, productive lives." Smiling, you thank this doctor (this time meaning it) and go home to tell your family the happy news.

Sound comical? You were given identical information by each physician, yet one sounded like the voice of doom while the other sounded like a reprieve. Both physicians told you that the drug worked well 90% of the time and failed 10% of the time. Your impression, and perhaps your subsequent decision, depended not on *what* was said but *how* it was said.

Professionally trained decision makers are not immune to this trick. In a now-famous study, 167 doctors were divided into two groups. One group was told that 10% of people undergoing surgery for lung cancer would die during the surgery and that 66% would die within five years. The second group of doctors was told that 90% of these same patients would survive surgery and 34% would survive five years. The physicians were asked whether they would choose surgery for themselves if they had lung cancer. The surprising results: Significantly more doctors in the second group (those told that 90% of the patients would survive) chose surgery than did doctors in the first group. In other words, whether the physicians chose surgery for themselves depended not on the data, but on how the data were presented. So powerful is the method of data presentation that even physicians need to be wary.

How we initially perceive reality, therefore, depends on the language used to describe it. But the problem does not stop there, since we are also profoundly affected by old assumptions and viewpoints.

Don't be ruled by language.

IT'S ALL IN HOW YOU FRAME IT

"Is it better to be killed or better to die?"
—Surgeons' saying

No one can live for very long without gathering a collection of personal assumptions and viewpoints about how the world works. These assumptions are usually helpful, enabling us to respond to new situations and to make decisions in the face of uncertainty. Sometimes, however, they do not quite fit reality and may lead us astray. This type of pitfall has been extensively studied by social scientists, who have coined the term *framing* to indicate the act of forming specific assumptions or viewpoints. We discussed the importance of frames earlier; now let's explore the profound effect that framing can have upon our interpretation of information and upon our decisions.

Suppose, for example, that you have a tumor in your neck, and that your physician tells you that your chance of dying from the tumor is about 8% if untreated. Luckily, surgical removal of the tumor is quite possible, but would leave you with a long scar across your face. Many people would accept the scar as a reasonable price to pay to avoid an almost 10% chance of death.

Now suppose that instead of having a tumor, you were born with a facial scar that provoked other children to make fun of you when you were growing up, and to this day attracts awkward stares from strangers. Suppose that a new plastic surgery had been developed recently that would rid you of the scar, but the chances of dying from the surgery were 8%. After some thought, many people would bravely choose to better their lives by deciding to have the surgery.

The difference between these two situations lies in their framing. In the first case, our minds are impressed with the fear of cancer, so that a cosmetic blemish seems a fair price to pay for safety. In the second case, our minds are set with the stigma of a deformity so emotionally painful that we would brave death to be released from its grasp. Different framing has led to different decisions, even though the risks were the same.

But how can both decisions be correct? Although we might understand these differences in terms of frames, the fact remains that these two situations are identical, and yet we paradoxically make different decisions in each. In one case, we choose a scar to avoid an 8% risk of death; in the other, we choose an 8% risk of death to avoid a scar. How can both seem so reasonable?

Here is another example of this type of paradox. The quote that started this section—"Is it better to be killed or better to die?"—is often cited by surgeons while deciding whether to offer surgery to a desperate patient when the result will probably be death. Although the remark seems flippant, it is far from a callous insensitivity born from too many hours on call. The question is important: When the treatment is just as likely to kill as the disease, how do surgeons choose? Framed one way, we might feel compelled to fight death with all our means, even if the chances are slim, since there is always the possibility of victory. Hope springs eternal. Framed another way, we might think it better to let nature take its course, sparing our patients the agony of treatment, even as we accept defeat without trying. The question is one for ourselves: Should we risk killing our patients while fighting for them, or should we let death take its easy course with no chance of victory? Is it better to be killed or to die?

We cannot ignore our frames. Sure, it is important to know the tradeoffs and estimate their risks, and in fact these tasks are the first two steps of our own plan for decision making. But decisions cannot be made by consideration of objective facts alone, since the most important components of our decisions are different from person to person.

Although we cannot ignore our frames, we can change them. We can be aware of how we use our frames to see the world. This requires us to change viewpoints, and to challenge our cherished assumptions. It is hard work, but worth it if we can avoid decisions we will later regret.

For example, when told that use of a drug has a 10% risk of death, we should not stop there; we have to turn it around the other way and remind ourselves that this means that there is a 90% survival rate. It is crucial to actively turn the data backward and forward, to see the same facts from as many viewpoints as you can imagine.

Likewise, we should give adequate time and intensity to contemplation of the meaning of our decisions. A second, or even third, examination of the meaning we place on the tradeoffs is often essential. What is really more important to us, avoidance of risk or physical appearance? Is getting rid of the scar really worth the risk of dying? Will I really be able to live with a permanent facial scar once the tumor is gone?

There are no right answers, and different people will choose differently. Intuition, beliefs, and gut feelings are useful guidelines here. Just be sure to examine all the different ways that the same data might be presented to you; no one else will.

Turn it upside down.

HOW MUCH INFORMATION IS ENOUGH?

I recently ran an Internet search on a few common diseases, just to see how much information was out there. "Breast cancer" has more than two million Web sites, "vitamins" has more than three million, and "stroke" has more than four million. Almost without exception, you will find similar numbers for almost any medical problem you choose.

There is no way that any one human being can visit all of these Web sites, much less absorb and evaluate all of the available information. And I'm not even counting the millions of medical articles and thousands of medical books that might be relevant to your needs.

So when do you stop looking for information? How do you know when you have enough? What if the very next article in the list contains the very cure you are seeking?

There are no cut-and-dried answers, of course. But there are some indications that you have exhausted most of what is out there. To begin with, for any one illness there is simply not enough information to fill millions of Web sites and articles without repetition. As you read more and more, you will find the same material again and again. At this point, you can feel fairly certain you have covered the basics.

You might feel tempted to read every article ever written about your topic. Perhaps you will find something rare and new that will show you a cure. But the more likely outcome is frustration as you attempt to read a vast and unorganized mass of data. It is better to limit your search to review articles in medical journals, to medical textbooks, and to a few reliable Web sites.

Because you don't want to get so bogged down in the research process that your decision becomes dangerously delayed, you can also usually restrict your search to sources appearing in the last two or three years. And remember that you don't have to see everything; the really good treatments are rarely hidden in some obscure journal. They will be repeated and broadcast throughout the medical literature.

On the other hand, if you are searching for something more specific, or if you need to find something truly different, don't be afraid of wading through oceans of medical articles and data. This task is easier than it once was, since the data are now organized on the Internet in sites such as PubMed. Use these sites, and learn to use the search engines; the results will be worth it. With these indispensable tools, the days of looking for obscure references for hours in the library are just about over. And don't forget to use your doctors; they can guide you to new sources of information and can highlight treatments you may not have noticed.

So how do you know when enough is enough? When do your efforts reach the point of diminishing returns? When the information you are reading begins to be repetitive, and when you get a sense that you are familiar with the current thinking in the field.

You'll know when enough is enough.

WHAT IF THERE AREN'T ANY NUMBERS?

Occasionally a medical problem is so rare or so poorly understood that there are no reliable numerical estimates of the success of treatment or the degree of risk to be found in the medical literature. You might find that your particular type of leukemia is mentioned only in a few paragraphs in a few articles, or that the specific combination of medicines you are taking for asthma is not mentioned anywhere in the textbooks. You may be up against a gap of knowledge.

Medical reviews will never admit ignorance so bluntly, but you can tell this is the case if the available numbers are based on only a few patients or if there are only a few studies. And you can detect medical ignorance if none of the experts agree. If the success of a treatment of ovarian cancer is 10% in one article, 85% in another, and 40% in a third, it may be that no one knows the right answer.

Your job as a decision maker just got harder, for now you have no quantitative barometer to help you choose among critical options.

In these cases, I think it is best to give up our hopes of finding data fit for interpretation. We must admit that medical knowledge is incomplete, even though this admission is frightening and discomforting when our well-being hangs in the balance. Where then can we turn when there are no data in the literature or on the Internet to guide our decisions?

We have to turn to people. Even the most rare and difficult of diseases is treated by *some* doctor *somewhere*, and that experience makes this person an expert. His or her knowledge might be imperfect and may not be published in the medical literature, but it is there nevertheless and may be just what you need. The best thing is then to seek out the doctors with experience with your problem, and to rely on these experts whether you find them in your hometown or half a world away. Be encouraged, since the experts have the most experience with these illnesses and their insight is often confirmed when the scientific studies are finally done.

Get help if there aren't any numbers.

Timing Isn't Everything

Eddie B. is a 21-year-old college student who has had asthma all his life. Although not life threatening, his breathing difficulties have limited his participation in sports and often keep him at home when he would rather be with friends or at school. He recently read an article about a new medication for asthma that reported complete and long-lasting relief of asthma 95% of the time. "Wow," he thought, "This might be just the thing!" He searched for more information about the drug, finding articles that were a bit less rosy; one reported a success rate of 65%, another discussed some complications, and a third showed some unpleasant interactions between this new medication and other asthma drugs that Eddie used. After mulling it over for a few weeks, Eddie's first impression remained strong and he went to his doctor and all but demanded a prescription for the new medication.

Mary Q. discovered she had colon cancer not long ago. Realizing the serious nature of this problem, she and her family have traveled to several major cancer centers across the country to determine where she will receive her medical care. Each center had many impressive features as well as some disadvantages. Although the fourth center she visited was more than five hundred miles from her home, she was so impressed by what she saw that she made her decision to stay there on the very afternoon of her visit.

Both Eddie and Mary have allowed their medical decisions to be affected by the order in which they received their information. In Eddie's case, his first impression of the success rate of the new medication was so strong that he virtually ignored the other, less glowing reports by the time he came to his decision several weeks later. Psychologists call this the *primacy effect*; first impressions are hard to shake. As in Eddie's case, this effect can be more powerful if the decision occurs later, allowing the second impressions to fade away with time.

Mary, by contrast, made her decision immediately before she had left her fourth center. Had she gone home first, the immediacy of this center might have paled somewhat, allowing her to consider all the centers equally. Psychologists have a name for this effect, too, calling it the *recency effect*; last impressions are the most vivid and can be the most influential, especially if decisions are made immediately.

You want to avoid being influenced by either the primacy or recency effect, since your success with a medical treatment will have nothing to do with the order in which you receive information. One way to do this is to keep a list of all the options and review it periodically, so that no one option is ever even halfway forgotten. In other words, you want to blunt your first impressions. Another tip is to delay making your decisions, even if ever so slightly, so that you have an opportunity to review all the options equally and avoid being unduly influenced by the option you have seen most recently. And as always, being aware of these influences is more than half the battle.

First or last may not be best.

—THE MATHEMATICS AND STATISTICS OF DECISION MAKING—

Most normal people dread mathematics and are bored by statistics. But as patients, we quickly find these unpleasant subjects forced upon us by necessity, since medical truths are expressed in the language of percentages. Don't expect to be told that an operation will cure you; expect instead to be told that the chances of success are better than 80%. In this new language of medicine, our fates are wrapped in percentages.

We must therefore learn this language of numbers so that we can interpret what we read and learn about our medical circumstances. Although you could skip this section and still benefit from our six steps of medical decision making, I would recommend that you at least skim this material and perhaps reread it later. I promise to make these lessons as mathematically painless as possible.

HOW TO INTERPRET PERCENTAGES

Many people are convinced that doctors have a secret language, a way of saying things to themselves that only they can understand. And many doctors firmly deny the existence of such a language, with the exception of some admittedly overblown jargon. Well, if the truth be known, there really is a secret language, and it really is used by doctors every day, and it really is hidden from most patients. But it is not a language of glamorous innuendo or scientific inspiration. It is the language of plain old mathematics, of drab percentages and dry numbers.

How can that be? Why would anyone try to distill the exciting nuances of medicine into mere numbers? The answer lies in considering what is important in medical decisions, what constitutes the meat of medical thinking: it is the ability to evaluate medical treatment and the ability to assess risk. Doctors are not content to know that a new operation cures gallbladder disease most of the time, they want to know more. They want to know exactly how often the operation works—does it work 60% of the time or 98%? And they are not content to know that the risk of the operation is low. They want to know just how low—is it 1% or 10%? These differences can mean life or death for their patients, and like it or not, these differences can only be expressed as percentages. And so you have it: Numbers are the heart and soul of medical thinking.

Look at some of the medical data you have struggled so hard to find and you will see what I mean. Numbers are everywhere. Medical textbooks talk about incidence and prevalence of certain diseases, and medical articles show you rates of efficacy and safety; these are all percentages. Even the casual television news item will often quote an encouraging rate of success. Like a floating iceberg, the language of mathematics bobs just beneath the surface of medicine.

Obviously, then, we must learn this language of numbers and grasp the meaning of percentages if we are to make good medical decisions. But as anyone who has ever taken a math class can tell you, the problem is that the interpretation of numbers can be tough. Numbers can be slippery, and we are easily fooled by complex ways of data presentation even when medical authors do their best to make their ideas clear.

My goal here is to show you how to speak this secret language of doctors, how to think about percentages when you are struggling to evaluate a new medication or assess the risk of a surgery. (For those of you who have always hated math, take heart; the language is not too difficult, and you might even find its application to medical matters interesting.) We will start by looking at some straightforward percentages and then build intuition for the more difficult examples.

50:50. What does it mean to say that a medication has a 50% chance of working? The easiest analogy is that of a coin toss; if you take this medicine, it will work with the same chance of a flipped coin landing heads. And the same is true for percentages close to 50%; a medication with a 45% chance of success works just a little less often than a coin toss, and that with a 55% chance works just a little more often. So far, so good; let's go on to the next percentage.

30%. Thirty percent is about one-third, so to say that a surgery has a 30% risk of complications means that something bad will happen one out of three times. Door number one, door number two, or door number three. . . .

10%. Suppose your doctor tells you that the chances of dying or being seriously injured by an operation are low—say about 10%. How can we understand this risk with the same intuition with which we grasp 50% as a coin toss?

Here's a thought experiment that may help. Imagine that your best friend is hosting a dinner party for nine of his closest friends. All ten of you are seated at the dinner table, about to begin the first course, a delicious bowl of hearty pea soup. Try to visualize your particular group of friends; it may help to write down a list. After the soup course, your friend hurries in from the kitchen to tell you that he is sorry, but he has made a terrible mistake. He has unintentionally mixed poison in one of the soup bowls. One of the guests will die.

After recovering from the shock, you reflect that your risk of dying from the soup is the same as the risk of complications from your planned operation, about a 1 in 10 chance. And later (assuming you survive), it dawns on you that this unnerving dining experience can be used to test your willingness to accept a 10% risk of any medical treatment: You can say that the treatment and its risks are acceptable to you if you would be willing to have dinner with your friend in order to obtain the benefits of the treatment, i.e., if you would eat the peas to beat the disease.

A nice aspect of this test is that it lets you think about a 10% risk in concrete terms that are personal and specific to you, much as using the idea of a coin toss helps to think about a risk of 50%. The idea of attending a dinner party for ten in which one guest is sure to die may be terrifying to you, outweighing the benefits promised by the medical treatment under consideration. Or conversely, ten people may seem like a large enough group to you that you are willing to bet that you will not be the unlucky guest receiving the poisoned soup, especially if the benefits of treatment allow you to avoid an even greater risk. Again, there are no right answers, only ways of thinking.

Percentages Less than 1%. Watch out for these. Small percentages are both common and treacherous because the human mind is simply not built to understand the differences between two small numbers. Let's see why.

Suppose you are a passenger on an airplane, and the pilot announces that your risk of dying from a crash that day is 1 in 800,000. That might seem comforting; 800,000 is such a large number that it would take you more than nine days working around the clock just to count that high. But what if I told you that the usual risk of dying on a flight was 1 in 8,000,000, ten times less than the flight you are on? You can see the problem. It is as if our brains only have one concept for "very small," so that we perceive two very small risks as intuitively identical, even though one might be ten times the other.

If the percentages are not excessively tiny, there are ways to gain intuition for what they mean. For example, a risk of 2% can be thought of as the risk of dying from the pea soup at a dinner party for fifty, and the risk of 1% can be had by attending a party for one hundred. Or you can think of a risk of 1% as just a little more than the chances of flipping a coin heads seven times in a row. But for smaller percentages—for huge dinner parties and countless coin flips—the numbers begin to blur in our imaginations and we lose intuition.

So remember that small is small, and that tiny differences may not much matter. The risk of taking one medication for gout might be ten times that of another, but if the risk of the first is 0.1% and the risk of the second is 0.2%, they are virtually the same and your choice might be best determined by cost rather than safety. In most cases, you will have to rely on the individual circumstances to make your decision.

Let's now go the other way and look at large percentages.

75%. Even if we believe that a 75% risk is manageable, it is the same risk as attending our dinner party with four guests and three bowls of poisoned soup. I would be nervous....

Percentages Greater than 99%. We have the same problem for risks such as 99.999% as we did for very small risks; our brains are not equipped to grasp the small differences between large percentages. Just as we have only one conception of "very small," we seem to have only one conception of "close to certainty." So don't be too upset if the doctor says your chances are 99.9% and you were hoping for 99.999%; the differences are too small to imagine.

Look at numbers with concrete examples.

PITFALLS AND SPECIAL CIRCUMSTANCES OF PERCENTAGES

Success as the Flip-Side of Failure

This is a common trap, as we discussed earlier in It's All in How You Say It (page 112). Remember that a success rate of 85% is equivalent to a failure rate of 15%, and that how these rates are presented may color your decisions. The moral of the story is to always, always, *always* turn success rates into failure rates and failure rates into success rates.

Weighty Consequences

Our interpretation of risk is naturally altered by the potential consequences of our decisions. In our dinner party experiment, for example, how would our decision process be altered if the poison was not lethal, but merely induced some mild nausea for a few minutes? In that case, a 10% or even a 50% risk might seem very acceptable indeed.

On the other hand, sometimes we ignore the consequences of a decision if the risk is low. If we are told that a certain operation is associated with a 5% risk of dying, we might find ourselves agreeing easily to the operation, since 5% is so small. I think that what commonly happens here is that since the thought of our own death is so frightening and unacceptable, we gloss over a small percentage of risk to ourselves, thinking something like "it can't and won't happen to me." But when you think of a 5% risk as equivalent to attending one of my dinner parties with only twenty people, it is perhaps not as low as we might want.

The moral: Pay close attention to the consequences of the decisions. Numbers alone are not everything.

Relative Risks: Size Matters

You will often want to compare the success rates of two treatments or compare their risks. Sometimes this information is given to you directly, as when you are given the success rate of each of the treatments individually. Other times you will be given a *relative rate*, as when drug A is reported to be 1.5 times more effective than drug B, or operation C has twice as much risk as operation D.

It would seem at first glance that your decision should be a no-brainer: Choose drug A and operation D. The unfortunate truth, however, is that relative risks are deceptive, and you really cannot make good decisions without knowing the *absolute* risks. Suppose, for example, that drug B had only a 20% chance of working. Then the advantage factor of 1.5 enjoyed by drug A translates to a 30% chance of success for drug A. If drug A had bad side effects or was painfully expensive, it might be a reasonable decision to turn down the rather modest gain in efficacy (from 20% to 30%) achieved by the use of drug A. On the other hand, if the success rate of drug B is 65%, the success rate of drug A becomes 98%. In this case, use of drug A would be almost a sure bet and would be hard to turn down.

Likewise, your preference for operation D might be affected by the absolute risk of operation C. If the risk of D was 5%, the risk of C would be only 10%; if the risk of D was 20%, then operation C would have a rather frightening risk of 40%. The difference between 10% and 40% would give most people pause for thought.

The moral: Relative risks are treacherous. *Always* demand to know the absolute risks.

Yearly Risks

You are in your doctor's office, and you are told that your chances of having a heart attack are about 4% per year unless you begin a new medication that is both difficult to find and expensive. Exactly how bad is 4% per year?

At first, you might think that this risk is trivial, since 4% is fairly small. But then you realize that this risk occurs *each year.* If you are 40 years old, this could represent an 80% chance of a heart attack by the time you are 60 years old. Seems high. . . .

But it's not that easy. For mathematical reasons, yearly percentages don't add up in a simple way. Here's why: You are really interested in the probability of *not* having a heart attack until you are 60 years old. The chances of *not* having a heart attack are 96% (100 − 4) each year. Multiplying 0.96 by itself 20 times (60 − 40 years) gives the probability of *not* having a heart attack at age 60; subtracting the result from 1.0 (100%) gives the probability of having at least one heart attack during this time.

The bottom line of all of this math is that the risk of a heart attack by the age of 60 for our patient is 56%, not the 80% that we had thought. This difference is significant, although it may or may not influence your decision. The point is that percentages do not directly add up over long periods. (This argument also solves the paradox of a risk of 104% arising after 26 years from a risk of 4% per year.)

The moral: The risk of yearly percentages over a long period of time is less than what simple addition would suggest.

THE MYTH OF ZERO RISK

A common scenario facing patients is being told that the risk of a treatment such as an operation or blood transfusion is very small but not zero. No matter how small the risk may be, most people find this unsettling, and they may inappropriately alter their decisions to eliminate the risk completely. In this fashion, many patients have denied themselves needed medications or operations out of fear of what is really an extremely small risk. This phenomenon was coined the "enchanting appeal of zero risk" in a fascinating article by epidemiologist and physician Donald Redelmeier that examines different ways patients can be misled into poor decisions.

There are at least two ways out of this trap. One is to realize that, in fact, absolute zero risk can never be achieved in the real world. There is always a small, but non-zero, chance of disaster in anything we do. That's just life.

The other more tangible way to cope with this is once again to compare the risk of the treatment in question with the risk of something more familiar in everyday life. For example, if the risk of contracting severe hepatitis from taking a particular medication was said to be about 1 in 800,000, you would know that this compares with the risk of dying in a plane crash, as we pointed out earlier. Assuming you were relatively comfortable with flying, these considerations might make taking the medication more acceptable to you. More interesting numerical yardsticks pointed out by Redelmeier are the chances of dying in a single automobile trip (1 in 1,000,000), and the chance of living more than 100 years (1 in 20,000).

Since everything we do at every moment of our day carries a small risk of disaster, it is useful to gain an intuitive feel for what a small risk means. The best way to do this is by comparison with common everyday events.

No risk is a zero risk.

STATISTICS MADE EASY

There is more to medical statistics than percentages, of course, since many problems arise when trying to describe medical facts with numbers. One such problem is that the success rates and estimates of risk that you read in a medical article are only approximations to reality. Even though a report might state that a drug is effective in 55% of the patients, the true rate of success might be larger or smaller. The study might have used a weak batch of the drug, or the patients tested might have been less healthy than most, or there might have been any number of differences in other variables. The percentages we read are only good guesses.

This means we have a problem when we want to compare two treatments. If one is said to be 55% effective and the other is said to be 68% effective, are they, in fact, different? Is the apparent difference in success rate real, or is there a difference simply because 68% is a guess that is too high and 55% is a guess that is too low?

This is the fundamental task of medical statistics: to tell us when the success rates or risks of two treatments are truly different. And this is also your fundamental task, since you want to pick the treatment that truly has the best chance of working and the least risk.

Statisticians have developed elaborate and complex mathematical methods to settle these questions. These methods are difficult to master and are not always effective, but the basic ideas are straightforward and the language used is universal among doctors. Fortunately, the language is surprisingly easy, as we will see.

The way in which doctors indicate that two percentages are really, truly different from one another is to say that the difference is *significant*. The word "significant" means something very specific in this language and indicates more than a vague importance. "Significant" means that a statistical test has been applied to the data, and that the two percentages are really different as judged by that test. A "significant" difference means that the difference is grade A, approved, and certified.

But knowing that the success rate of drug A is better than that of drug B is only half the battle, since we must also pay attention to the percentages themselves. For example, it might happen that the success rates of these two drugs are closely matched, say 84% for drug A and 83% for drug B. Even if this difference of 1% is significant in the statistical sense, it is so small that you might consider other factors (such as side effects or cost) in your choice of medication.

You might also read that a difference was not significant, or that it only approached significance. A medical study might report, for example, that operation A was associated with a 10% risk of death, whereas operation B had a 15% risk of death. If the authors state that the difference only approached significance, they mean that although the differences were intriguing, they cannot say for sure if one operation is more risky than the other. The 10% and 15% risks are estimates only, and it would be dangerous to conclude that operation B is really more risky than operation A based on these guesses.

Statisticians have helped doctors evaluate significance by calculating a number that measures how significant a difference is. This is called the "p value," and is typically a small number such as .01 or .05. When statisticians say that the difference between success rates of two treatments is "significant at the $p = .05$ level," they mean that the chances of being wrong—the chances of the difference not truly being significant—are less than 5%. Similarly, "significant at the $p = .01$ level" means that the chance of the difference *not* being significant is less than 1%. Small values of p are more powerful because small values indicate that our chances of being mistaken are less. Most doctors accept a p value of .05 as being adequate to conclude that there is a real difference, and many articles will report the p value explicitly.

There is much more to medical statistics, of course, enough to fill many careers. Many statistical tests are complex and require interpretation beyond the skill of most doctors. But as you read through medical articles, look for statements about significance. This is the language that will indicate the real significance of the data at hand.

"Significant" is significant.

HOW TO EVALUATE A MEDICAL TEST

Mary E. is a 48-year-old woman who has discovered a lump in her breast and is terrified at the thought of having breast cancer. Her doctor tells her that a biopsy will settle the issue, but that a new noninvasive test is available using MRI that does not require surgery. This new test is "just as good" as a biopsy and can be done in about an hour. Although Mary would like to avoid a biopsy if possible, she knows that the possibility of breast cancer is not to be taken lightly. Her doctor tells her that the new test is "95% accurate." But as comforting as that figure sounds, Mary realizes that she doesn't quite know what "95%" means. She does some reading about medical tests, finding a morass of intricate mathematical detail that seems as unfriendly as it is unhelpful. Let's see if we can shed some light on this difficult topic.

True and False, Positive and Negative. Evaluation of a medical test is more complicated than you might at first think. We are certainly interested in how well the test detects cancer, as this information will guide us to potentially lifesaving treatment. But it is just as important to know how well the test tells us when we do *not* have cancer. After all, it would be devastating to undergo surgery based on the results of this test, only to find later that there was no cancer at all. Tests must accurately tell us both when we do and when we do not have disease if they are to be trusted.

There are four possibilities to consider.

1. The test can correctly detect cancer when cancer is indeed present (the so-called true positive).
2. The test can wrongly detect cancer when no cancer is present (*false positive*).
3. The test can wrongly fail to detect cancer when cancer is in fact present (*false negative*)
4. The test can correctly fail to detect cancer when in fact there is no cancer at all (true negative).

Four possibilities, each described by a separate percentage; matters are getting complicated quickly.

Sensitivity and Specificity. Doctors try to simplify their thinking by using two calculations. The first is called the *sensitivity* of a test, and is simply the percentage at which the test detects cancer when cancer is in fact present; in other words, how well the test detects cancer. Using the language of the previous paragraph, the sensitivity is the number of true positives divided by the sum of the true positives and the false negatives, i.e., the number of times the test detects cancer divided by the number of times cancer is truly present, regardless of test results. A sensitivity of 60% means that the test will be positive in 60% of cases in which there is truly cancer. If you forget how sensitivity is calculated, remember that it measures how well the test detects cancer.

The second calculation is the *specificity* of a test. This index measures the ability of the test to exclude cancer when in fact cancer is absent, or in other words, how well the test detects the *absence* of cancer. It is calculated as the number of true negatives divided by the sum of the true negatives and false positives, i.e., the number of times the test excludes cancer divided by the number of times cancer is truly absent, regardless of test results. A specificity of 60% means that the test will be negative in 60% of the cases in which cancer is absent. If you forget how specificity is calculated, remember that it measures how well the test correctly excludes cancer.

A test can be sensitive without being specific and vice versa. For example, suppose a certain lab assay turned out to be positive for all women. The sensitivity of this assay as a test for breast cancer would be near 100%, since every woman with breast cancer would test positive. The specificity would be quite low (and the test would be useless), as the test would be incapable of excluding those women without breast cancer.

We must therefore look at both the sensitivity and specificity of a test, since both must be high if the test is to be useful. This task is a bit cumbersome, since neither of these indices tells the full picture by itself.

Values and Ratios. To help simplify matters further, two other indices are commonly used that provide a more intuitive evaluation of the test. The first is the *positive predictive value*, defined as the probability of cancer being present if the test is positive (this is calculated as the number of true positives divided by the sum of the true positives and false positives). This index captures what we really want to know about the test: If a patient tests positive, how likely is it that cancer is really present? Positive predictive value is useful in practice, although it can be unreliable if the disease in question is rare.

The second index used is the *likelihood ratio*, which measures how much more likely a positive test will be found in a patient with cancer when compared with a patient without cancer. It is calculated by dividing the sensitivity by (1 – specificity). If the likelihood ratio of a test is 2, for example, then patients testing positive will be twice as likely to have breast cancer as those who do not.

We can see now that Mary must be told more if she is to evaluate this new test for breast cancer. When her doctor says the test is "95% accurate," does he mean sensitivity? That would be nice, but how often will the test indicate a need for surgery when in fact she doesn't have cancer at all? Does he mean specificity? That would also be nice, but what is the chance of the test missing her cancer altogether? Or does her doctor mean the positive predictive value, harder to understand but more meaningful?

How can we use this information to evaluate a new diagnostic test?

Remember that any new test must be compared against older and more standard tests. If we are to trust the new MRI test for breast cancer, we must know how it compares with the tried and true methods.

Look for both a high sensitivity and specificity. If one of these indices is low, there are serious problems with the test.

Look for a high positive predictive value and a high likelihood ratio. These indices measure how we use the test in practice.

Realize that evaluation of a test is tricky business. Knowing the language of statistics will help your thinking, but don't hesitate to rely on your doctors for guidance.

Medical tests are like spouses; good ones are both sensitive and specific.

MORE TESTS: BACKWARD AND FORWARD

Let me point out one final pitfall in the interpretation of medical tests, building on what we just learned. Sooner or later, you will come across this problem in your reading.

Suppose you read that 95% of people with colon cancer were found to have a positive Lattice test (whatever a Lattice test is). The study used a large number of patients and seemed to be well constructed. You could therefore depend on the Lattice test as a good test for colon cancer. Right?

Wrong. This study showed that *if* you have colon cancer, you are likely to have a positive Lattice test. What we want to know is the reverse: *If* I have a positive Lattice test, how likely am I to have colon cancer? And the study doesn't answer that at all.

Let's look at this with another example. It is likely that 95% of all those having colon cancer can spell the word "cat," or in other words, *if* I have colon cancer, I am likely to be able to spell "cat." But that doesn't mean that the ability to spell simple words is a good test of colon cancer, because the reverse is not true: It is not true that *if* I can spell "cat," then I have a 95% chance of having colon cancer.

This may seem like a technical point, but it is worth remembering. An awareness of this difficulty may be useful to you as you read about various medical tests, and will guide you as you decide which tests to believe and which to discard.

Trees moving do not cause the wind.

WHAT HAPPENS FOR TWO EVENTS?

George B. is a 68-year-old executive with a serious heart problem that began several years ago with a heart attack. The resulting scar in his heart has caused a life-threatening alteration in his heart rhythm. His doctors have offered an operation that has a 75% chance of being successful, but George will need to take certain medications forever. Furthermore, the chances that those medications will preserve George's life after the surgery are 80%. Based on these two numbers, George concludes that his overall chances of doing well are between 75 and 80%. What would you tell him?

We all know intuitively that it is more difficult to be lucky twice than to be lucky once. Lottery winners do not expect to win again, and lightning rarely strikes twice. The same thinking applies to medical events, so that it is less likely that two treatments will be successful than each individually. Let's look at the mathematics in George's case to see why.

George is hoping that his operation will be successful, and he knows that the chances of this are 75%. He is also hoping that he is among the 80% of patients for whom the medications will work. The chances of both of these treatments being successful—the chances of his surgery being a success and of the medicine working—is not calculated by adding the two percentages, or taking their average, or taking the largest one. Unfortunately, we must multiply the two percentages to calculate the chances of both the surgery and the medication being successful. I say unfortunately because a multiplication of two percentages always yields a lower percentage than our starting point. In George's case, his chance of doing well is 0.75 x 0.80 = 0.60, or 60%. George needs to know about this reduced success rate if he is to make a wise decision.

It is difficult to be lucky twice.

WHEN THERE ARE MULTIPLE OPTIONS

See how you do on the following test. You must do it all in your head without writing anything down.

Bob has a 1985 red Camaro that is bigger than George's white Lexus. George's car is brand-new, but is smaller than Henry's black sedan. Henry has an antique sports car that is bigger than the Camaro.

What is the order of the cars by size from largest to smallest?

If you said sports car, Camaro, Lexus, you were correct. But right or wrong, you have to admit it wasn't all that easy to hold all these details in your mind. That is exactly what we must do when thinking about more than two medical options, except that the details are usually far more complex. We must remember which option is most effective and which is safest, and rank them in order of preference.

Examples are common in medicine. You might need to compare three different medicines used in the treatment of diabetes. Or you may have a choice of surgery, radiation therapy, chemotherapy, or some combination of these. And so on.

Because medical options are so much more important than ranking cars, I recommend that you make your job easier by writing everything down. Write down the success rates and the complication rates of each of the options as you learn about them, and your comparison later will be all the easier. This may seem like obvious advice, but taking notes is usually not the first thing that comes to mind when you are discussing a critical decision with your doctor.

Writing down the options is only a first step, since comparing three or more options contains some hidden subtleties. You would think that such a comparison would be straightforward, much like a wrestling match. Simply compare the options, one pair at a time, until a winner is declared. In the case of cancer, for example, one might compare surgery with radiation, radiation with chemotherapy, and chemotherapy with surgery. Then choose the winner.

Surprisingly, real life cheats us out of this simplicity. For there are circumstances in which surgery would be preferable to radiation, radiation preferable to chemotherapy, and yet chemotherapy preferable to surgery! It would be as if a wrestling tournament were held in which Bruno defeated Fritz, Fritz defeated Joe, and Joe defeated Bruno. How could this happen, and how would we choose?

To see how this odd state of affairs might arise, suppose that the success rate of surgery was 40%, that of radiation was 50%, and that of chemotherapy was 60%. And let's suppose that chemotherapy was likely to cause pain and kidney failure (even if it worked), that radiation was likely to cause pain but no kidney failure, and that surgery was unlikely to lead to complications. (Are you writing this down?)

In this case, you might prefer surgery to radiation to avoid pain, arguing that the efficacy of surgery and radiation were similar (the difference being only 10%). Similarly, you might prefer radiation to chemotherapy to avoid kidney failure. But you also could reasonably prefer chemotherapy to surgery since the 60% rate of success was so much better than 40%, regardless of the complications. Surprisingly, there is no obvious winner.

Although these circumstances may seem contrived, they occur in real life often enough to have drawn attention from decision theorists, who have labeled this state of affairs as *intransitivity*. Whatever the name and for whatever reason, it can be difficult to pick the best of several different options. As in this example, you can find yourself going around and around in a circle, always making comparisons but not coming up with a winner.

There are several ways off of this circle.

Write everything down. When you write things down, you can see all the options side by side. Then you can see all the statistics at once, just as you see all the prices on the shelves at the grocery store.

Compare all your options. Comparing *pairs* of options is useful but can sometimes fail to give a clear answer. You may need to compare all the options without breaking them into pairs. Be especially aware of this possibility if the numbers become confusing.

Factor in the meaning of each option. Many times the success rate or complication rate alone does not capture what it is about each option that is important to you. For example, your choice might be different if failure meant that a plastic surgery failed to make you look better, rather than if failure meant death. In these cases, it is the meaning that each option has for you that is likely to be the key factor. We will say more about this in chapter ten.

Choices get complicated. Write them down.

NINE

Step 5: Gathering Your Beliefs

"Belief is powerful. Ask the doctors."
—Father Frank Shore, in *The Third Miracle*

WE ALL HAVE BELIEFS. Some are true, some are false, but all of them help us understand the world around us. More than that, our beliefs shape how we perceive new information and how we respond to new situations. Beliefs about medicine are indeed very powerful, at times lifting our spirits but at other times dashing our reason. Even priests, experts in belief, know that some of the strongest examples of living beliefs are those routinely witnessed by doctors.

We will consider two types of beliefs in this chapter. The first are personal beliefs about medical expectations and our role as decision makers. These must be understood, and even challenged, if we are to achieve our full potential as medical decision makers. The second type of beliefs that we will discuss are those concerning data. These govern our ideas about what information we believe to be true, and what we reject. It doesn't matter how we arrived at these beliefs, or how long we've held them; what matters is that they are now an intrinsic part of who we are. Clearly, such beliefs affect every aspect of our medical decisions.

—PERSONAL BELIEFS—

WHAT DO YOU BELIEVE? AND WHY?

Why do we believe the things that we believe? Is it because we only believe what is proven to be absolute fact, or do we believe only what might seem to be true? How often are our beliefs false?

Social psychologists and philosophers have argued about these questions for years, so don't expect to come to any final answers. But we can at least be aware of the factors shaping our beliefs. These include our past experiences which have given us hundreds if not thousands of examples of how the world works and how it doesn't. Our education is an important factor, as are the opinions told to us by friends and family. What we read in newspapers or books and see on television is also influential, whether fact or fiction. In the end, all of this information is blended by our minds to form our own personal set of beliefs.

An interesting aspect of many of our beliefs is that they would turn out to be flat wrong if they could be evaluated by an all-knowing examiner. Since nobody can be right about everything, it follows that each of us must harbor some beliefs that are false. And for many issues (the presence of intelligent life on other planets, for example) there is simply not enough information available for us to know the truth beyond any shadow of a doubt. The result is that although many of our beliefs are based on clever intuition, many are simply guesses and some of them will inevitably be wrong.

Nor can we be right about each one of our medical beliefs. Some of these beliefs, such as the belief that the heart pumps blood to the body, are now so accepted and confirmed that it would be foolhardy to challenge them. Others, such as the assertion that taking large amounts of vitamin C prevents cancer, are only partly supported by data and are more controversial. And claims such as the assertion that moonbeams can heal wounds are probably completely false.

Why should we examine the way we form our beliefs? Because our beliefs determine how we interpret medical data, how we seek medical answers, and even what evidence our minds will admit. Each bit of information we obtain from our sources of medical information is subjected to this critical scrutiny based on our belief system, and only those that are consonant with our beliefs are kept for consideration. Our beliefs therefore act like a filter, letting in only the ideas that already make sense. And like an overprotective parent, our beliefs insulate us from new ways of thinking.

So what happens when we come across a medical idea or treatment that conflicts with our beliefs? We ignore this idea, even if it might have lifesaving merit. Only if our beliefs are flexible enough to be changed, and only if we are willing to change them, will we be able to make use of new information. That is why we must know which of our beliefs are irrevocable and which are really opinions that can be challenged.

Your beliefs are worth knowing.

WE SEE WHAT WE WANT TO SEE

I returned and saw under the sun that the race is not to the swift,
nor the battle to the strong, nor yet bread to the wise,
nor yet riches to men of understanding, nor yet favor to men of skill;
but time and chance happens to them all.

—Ecclesiastes

As you read medical literature and as you talk with your doctors, try to keep an open mind. Try to accept unpleasant facts even if you are hopeful for a good outcome. Try to judge the arguments in favor of medications even if you already want an operation. This may be the most difficult task in the world, for we all would rather accept pleasant beliefs than unpleasant realities. But it is reality that will have the last laugh, so keep an open mind.

But keeping an open mind is not always easy. The social psychologist Thomas Gilovich points out that people are notorious for being highly critical of unpleasant information that might threaten a pet theory. I see this often in my clinic when an optimistic family tells me that "well, every surgery has some risk" after I describe to them the very real risks of a proposed surgery that they have set their hearts on. Gilovich gives other examples from daily life. Most people believe that they themselves are smarter than others even though this cannot be universally true. Many professional gamblers explain their losses as mere flukes, thus justifying their persistent gambling. And studies have shown that football teams wearing unpleasant black uniforms are more likely to be penalized than those wearing more soothing colors. Even football referees find it difficult to be fair to the team in black.

An interesting example comes from the use of the drug laetrile, once touted as a cure for cancer. Despite careful studies showing that laetrile doesn't work, and despite the prohibition of the sale of laetrile in this country, numerous Web sites still extoll its virtues. I am sure that the true believers in laetrile find it difficult to read the articles showing it to be of no benefit. Perhaps they believe the truth is hidden by a government cover-up or trick. More interesting to me is my own difficulty reading their literature that explains why laetrile should work; knowledge of the scientific studies has made it difficult for me to keep an open mind. It is an uphill struggle to keep an open mind, requiring patience and balance.

So be skeptical. Be critical. And don't be afraid to consider evidence for what you do not want to believe.

Take off those rose-colored glasses.

JUDGING BOOKS BY THEIR COVERS

We all know that it is not wise to judge a book by its cover. Or at least, we think we do. Advertising agencies make millions of dollars each year because we forget this simple principle, proving that we are more likely to buy a product if it comes in a sleek and shiny box. Packaging makes a difference, even if we are wise to book covers.

This problem is a version of what is known as the *halo effect*, in which our judgment of an object is clouded by just one of its good qualities. An everyday example is our tendency to view physically attractive people as more capable, friendly, and worthy than people who are not so attractive. Admirable or not, this tendency has been verified by many studies of human behavior.

Unfortunately, the same pitfalls await us in medical decisions. Advertisements for drugs on television or in magazines are elegantly presented, appealing more to our senses and hopes than to our critical minds. The very shape of the pills you take and the boxes they come in seem more at home in a designer's studio than a pharmacy. And the same is true for medical personnel. The most charismatic, attractive physician may in fact know little of modern treatment, while a plain-looking, gruff doctor may know the very thing to save your life.

So don't be fooled by packaging. Look for the data supporting the drug you are considering or the operation you are planning. Look beyond the outward appearance and mannerisms of your physicians for true knowledge and competence. Don't judge a book by its cover.

Buy the contents, not the package.

BELIEFS IN WISHES AND CONTROL

Sandy K. is a 45-year-old executive who founded her own company ten years ago and continues as its CEO. Unfortunately, just as her business became lucrative, she developed severe rheumatoid arthritis affecting her hands, reducing her presence at work and preventing her from enjoying many of her favorite activities at home. Highly intelligent and demanding, she reviewed countless books and articles on arthritis while consulting with more than a few physicians specializing in this disease. Her medications are sophisticated and the schedules are complex, but her pain is only partly relieved and the arthritis seems to be relentlessly progressing.

The failure of her medications to restore her to normal bothered Sandy, and she found herself attending a local health fair even though she joked about "all that rip-off quackery" with her friends. There she found a booth selling a type of milk shake "loaded with trace elements, guaranteed to cure arthritis." The theory was that the trace minerals and elements mixed in with the milk shake were exactly what most people were missing in their diets and exactly what their bodies needed to "heal themselves." On the counter, a thick book was laid open to exhibit letters from customers who had been cured of their illness. After perusing the rest of the health fair, Sandy could not help but return to this booth to sign up for a year's supply of the stuff.

Why would a savvy, successful business woman like Sandy do that? What would compel her to purchase a year's worth of expensive supplies on the spur of the moment, based only on advertisements, unsubstantiated testimonials, and no scientific studies at all? Leaving aside the question of whether trace minerals can really cure arthritis, why would Sandy invest her personal resources based on evidence that she would never find acceptable for her business investments? And from a company that she hadn't investigated at all?

Let's not be too hard on Sandy; most of us would do the same. Despite intense efforts, modern medicine cannot cure Sandy, and, in fact, predicts her inexorable decline. Disappointment and fear smolder so much in the back of her mind that her wish for cure and relief of her symptoms is vivid enough to taste. This is the wish that clouds her normal skepticism and permits her to accept the claims of salesmen without criticism. She wants so much to be better that she is willing to believe anything.

I think there is an additional element that moves us in times like these, and that is the wish for control. You do not have to be a patient for too long before you realize that you are no longer in control of your life in the same way as before you became ill. As patients we must give up a certain amount of control to the doctor, following the "doctor's orders." But there is more; we find ourselves also at the mercy of nurses, X-ray technologists, phlebotomists, and stubborn insurance companies. "To be patient" in fact means to endure some amount of suffering without complaint, i.e., to surrender control of your comfort, at least temporarily. The resentment invoked is reflected in Ambrose Bierce's more honest definition of patience as "a minor form of despair, disguised as a virtue." Loss of control is especially difficult for aggressive executives such as Sandy who base their identities and self-esteem upon their ability to be in control at all times.

So for Sandy, taking the concoction she found at the health fair put her back in the driver's seat and offered her the security of control that she was missing. No more waiting for the doctor, no more following instructions of every technologist and nurse she encountered, no more being accountable for complex medicine schedules. She had control; she could melt away her pain whenever she liked. Or so she hoped.

Wishes can cloud our thinking and impair our assessment of dangerous risks. But it is good to have wishes, and normal to want to control the forces in our world. As human beings, we must accept the fact that we will all spend some of our energy wishing and some of our energy seeking control. But it is also human nature to make rational decisions. To do this we must acknowledge that some of our most cherished wishes may not be granted, and that many forces are simply beyond our control. It is the balance between these two aspects of human nature that gives rise to a good medical decision.

You can't always get what you want.

Beliefs in Happy Endings

I was never as strong, smart, and invulnerable as when I was 16 years old. I knew all the answers to life's questions, I understood all that there was in the world, and nothing bad would ever happen to me.

Until I turned 17, of course, and then it was downhill from there. We all learn this lesson as we age: We are not invulnerable, bad things can happen to us (and ultimately do), and much that happens to us is beyond our control. But although it is one thing to learn this gradually from a natural progression of life's array of bumps and knocks, it is entirely another to face these truths abruptly by confrontation with a serious medical problem.

Times of medical threat force us to face just how vulnerable we are and make us painfully intimate with our mortality and fragility. And yet paradoxically, many people somehow regain their teenage overconfidence and once again feel invulnerable. We might see a man facing open-heart surgery by denying that there were any risks at all, or we might hear of a woman refusing chemotherapy because she was certain that vitamins would cure her. Every physician has had the uncomfortable experience of treating a patient who will not consider all the available alternatives. It is as if there is comfort in the act of becoming overconfident, since our overconfidence tells us that everything will be okay.

But of course, that's not true, and bad things do indeed happen. Decision theorists tell us that one of the biggest mistakes made in all aspects of decision making is being overconfident. For overconfidence provides us comfort by turning our minds off, short-circuiting the skeptical and critical thinking so badly needed by those facing tough decisions.

So how can we fight this natural tendency to be overconfident? My suggestion is to make a strenuous attempt to challenge your own beliefs, to overthrow your own smug confidence. By actively thinking of all the reasons and all the possibilities why you might be wrong, you can free your mind to consider perspectives and alternatives that you could not consider before. Ask a good friend to play devil's advocate, to challenge your beliefs and assumptions. Strategies of this type have also been recommended by decision theorists, and have proven useful in fields other than medicine.

Kill overconfidence before it kills you.

BELIEFS IN MEDICINE

In the popular television series *ER*, we are taken inside the emergency room to witness heroic efforts of dedicated physicians as they implement the latest medical maneuvers to dramatically rescue the newest victim. We see these doctor-heroes perform intubations, insert chest tubes, crack chest walls, and prescribe a mind-boggling array of drugs as easily as we make an omelet. Successful or not, these actions are ordered rat-a-tat-tat by the doctors, who have obviously read and memorized the medical books. It is always clear what to do and when to do it.

But that's not how it is in real life. During my training, for example, after each busy night in the emergency room, we attended a mandatory meeting in a cramped and sweaty treatment room early the next morning. Bone-tired and huddled together in an intimate circle, each of us grimly listened in turn while an attending physician grilled us about our mistakes of the night before. There was always plenty to talk about, and the tone was rarely friendly.

You won't see this type of meeting on television, because the discussions are too revealing and too frightening. Should that patient have been intubated before the peritoneal lavage? Was that the right sequence of drugs? Why in the world wasn't that specific test ordered? Weren't we aware that a chest tube should have been placed much earlier? That we made mistakes and that they were revealed to all was frightening enough. But even more disturbing was that all too often we realized that there was not a perfect decision, even in retrospect. To be sure, the attending physician would have an opinion that he or she gladly shared with us. But in some cases there were simply no studies or data to support one decision over another. Or often the data were conflicting, with one article saying one thing and another saying the opposite.

I have tried to stress the importance of reading about your medical problems, of finding the alternatives available to you, and of discovering the best available estimates of efficacy and risk. But even if we have oceans of data and years of experience, the best medical path is often not obvious. A particular treatment for leukemia might be touted by one center and dismissed at another, or one article might praise a surgery while another condemns it. The best available medical information is still often incomplete, frequently vague, and sometimes downright contradictory. It will be of great help to seek advice from physicians who deal with these difficulties daily. But as you decide what information to believe and how to interpret the confusion, remember: Don't expect the moon from modern medicine.

We don't have all the answers.

BELIEFS ABOUT MORAL QUESTIONS

Morality was defined by Samuel Johnson to be "the doctrine of the duties of life," meaning that some of our acts are wrong and others right. Although it is not my intention or ability to discuss ethics and morality, it is true that most of us hold some beliefs of our place in the moral order of things. We have a sense of what we should do and of our duties to those around us. Although this moral sense is an important aspect determining how we approach medical decisions, it can at times collide with our other needs.

Consider Abbie H., for example, an 88-year-old woman requiring renal dialysis, who was recently discovered to have leukemia in addition to renal failure. The ordeal of dialysis alone would be more than enough for any one person, but the prospect of adding the discomfort of chemotherapy for leukemia was more than Abbie wanted to bear. Left to herself, she would have refused treatment and hoped for a painless death.

The problem was that Abbie had always been the leader of her family, their source of strength during hard times. Even though her two daughters and three sons were adults with families of their own, they still depended upon her for emotional and financial support. Abbie took this responsibility for her family seriously, so much so that her wish to refuse treatment provoked tearful guilt at the thought of "leaving my family defenseless." On the surface, her children had urged her to do what was right for herself, but in a subtle, almost subliminal way they had encouraged the dependence and guilt that prevented Abbie from making her final choice.

I don't have a good answer for what to do in case moral concerns conflict with your other decision considerations. On the one hand, I would encourage you to choose what seems right for you, even if it may not seem right for society or those around you. Ambrose Bierce might have agreed when he defined "moral" as that which conforms "to a local and mutable standard of right." And it also fits with the ideal of the importance of the individual.

On the other hand, it is clear that for some people, the concerns of others take primary importance and outweigh other considerations. The arguments can become a bit circular here, since the individual's most important concerns now become what seems right for others. But there is no denying that many people will choose as Abbie has chosen: to live as long as possible, even at the expense of her own comfort.

What I would recommend if you find yourself in this type of quandary is to clearly identify for yourself which of your tradeoffs are for those around you or for society and which are for yourself as an individual. This is not an easy task and may take some reflection. Like Abby, you will have to decide for yourself which of these is most important to you.

Be careful of ought and should.

CHALLENGE YOUR BELIEFS

"When someone challenges our beliefs,
it is as if someone criticized our possessions."
—Thomas Gilovich, *How We Know What Isn't So*

If you ran a large business, you would not want to be surrounded by people who always thought all of your ideas were wonderful. To the contrary, your most valuable employee would be one who would not be afraid to challenge your ideas, one who would force you to rethink your ideas again and again.

In a similar fashion, it is healthy to challenge your own assumptions as you mull over your medical decisions. The purpose is not to change your beliefs, since I am assuming that your beliefs about your own medical care will be pretty well justified in your mind. But it is good to periodically review the reasons for your beliefs, if only to feel more secure in holding them. And once in a while this exercise will teach us something new.

For example, if you believe your doctor is competent, ask yourself why. Because of recommendations from others and demonstrated medical knowledge, or because of his or her clothing? If you believe radiation is bad, why? What experience have you had that led to that fear? If you must have an operation this very month, ask why. What will change if you put it off? If you believe that a new medication will cause bad side effects, ask why. Is your belief based on medical articles or on what a friend told you? If you believe that you will not have complications from a particular operation, what leads you to that belief? Are you denying an unpleasant reality? If you believe that certain vitamins are worth buying because they will give you more energy, ask yourself why. Is it because the clerk at the store where you bought them said so? And if you believe that you ought to undergo a specific treatment for the sake of your family, ask why and for whom.

As you can see, this is not a very fun game. We take our beliefs personally, as Gilovich pointed out in the quote above. I am asking you to attack your own beliefs rather cruelly and with a degree of sharp criticism. But you can do this in the privacy of your own mind, with no pressure to share your thoughts with anyone, if you so choose. Again, the goal is not to get you to change your beliefs, but rather, to allow you to understand why you hold them as you do. You may find that some of your beliefs are based on facts and figures, while others cannot really be explained. It doesn't matter. The goal here is to understand your beliefs and to become more secure in them.

Be hard on yourself. It's safer than you think.

HOPE *VERSUS* REALITY

If I had to summarize my message to you thus far, I would say this: Be hard-nosed about what you believe, do not be fooled by flimflam or wishful thinking, and be very, very careful not to believe rubbish. If hard evidence says that your cancer will kill you in two years, arrange your affairs and make your peace rather than invest your time in magic crystals. If studies show that your diabetes is likely to cause blindness even with medication, accept the inevitable and make use of your time to see.

But life doesn't work that way, and neither do we, not completely. Even if all your reading and consulting and hard-nosed critical thinking has convinced you that your chances of succumbing to your illness are 90%, there is always hope that you will be among the lucky 10% who do well. As decision makers, I have tried to suggest that you choose your beliefs rationally. But as human beings, we are built in such a way that we cannot completely believe in our total misfortune, even if that event is almost certain. In our minds, hope indeed springs eternal.

But which should we believe? Is it best to resign ourselves to the fate ordained by studies and statistics, or do we hope for a more pleasant fortune, no matter how unlikely? I would suggest to you that we must do both. Regardless of the odds, we must have a foot in each camp: one in the camp of despair, and the other in the camp of hope. For this is the only way that we can be realistic about what might happen and still be faithful to our human quality of hope. It is a belief worth having.

And who knows; you might indeed be part of that lucky 10%. . . .

Let hope spring as eternal as it wants.

—BELIEFS ABOUT DATA—

We are bombarded by data every day and every hour and every second of our lives. The televisions in our living rooms, the newspapers on the tables, the advertisements on billboards—all of these hurl information at us wherever we are. We don't accept it all at face value, of course, since much of it is unreliable. But which data we ignore and which we choose to accept depends on our underlying beliefs about the world that may be so subtle that they escape awareness. The nature of these beliefs and how they influence our interpretation of medical data as we make our medial decisions is the subject of this section.

BELIEFS BASED ON COINCIDENCE: WHY WE KNOW WHAT ISN'T SO

One of the best lessons about beliefs was taught to me by a piece of sculpture at the Berkeley Art Museum in California. It was a hot summer afternoon, and I was lazing my way from one painting to another when I saw it, all by itself in a nook at the top of a wide stairway. It looked like a grandfather clock, tall and narrow, with a face at the top. But instead of numbers, the face was fitted with a hammer, pulled back and poised to strike a bell. Every so often, the hammer would be released by some hidden mechanism, and the bell would chime. On the floor in front of this clock-piece was a thick pad that looked like a foot switch, connected to the innards of the device by an electrical cable. I watched as a number of people tried stamping on the pad to get the hammer to strike, but to no avail. I decided to try myself, and after some trial and error, I found that a pattern of stamp-stamp-rest-stamp would make the hammer go. I backed away, secretly proud that I alone had solved the puzzle.

After exploring the rest of the museum, I returned to the clock-piece and for some reason decided to follow the electrical cable to see where it went and what it did. I was mortified to find that it ended in thin air behind the piece, not connected to anything at all. The hammer had been striking at random, not caring a whit about my pattern of stamps and rests.

In other words, my beautiful solution to the puzzle of the hammer was complete nonsense. I was seeing patterns that simply weren't there.

In his enlightening and entertaining book, *How We Know What Isn't So*, Thomas Gilovich shows us how often this fallacy appears in human thought. Over and over again, people have attempted to explain random coincidence by complex theories that turn out to be as wrong as they are appealing. And once believed, these theories just won't go away. An example is the widely held belief that infertile couples who adopt a child are more likely to conceive after the adoption; another is that more babies are born when the moon is full. Both of these beliefs have been intensively studied, both are completely false, and both are believed by millions.

Gilovich has studied one such belief in detail, the belief found among basketball players in "hot hands." This is the belief that once a basketball player has made a few successful baskets, he is more likely to score than if he had made no baskets at all. He is then on a roll, or as his teammates might say, "his hands are hot."

As intuitively appealing as this theory might be, it turns out to be false. Gilovich gives exhaustive and compelling evidence collected over a long period of time that "hot hands" simply do not exist. What really happens is that runs of successful shots are noticed more if they occur after a few successful baskets than if they occur with no warning. No matter if those runs are to be expected based on random chance alone. Someone notices this "connection," points it out to someone else, and *voilà*! "Hot hands."

Here's the really interesting part: Nothing can shake this belief. When professional basketball players and coaches were confronted with this incontrovertible proof that "hot hands" do not exist, they turned a deaf and hostile ear. The careful studies and arguments, scientifically and meticulously gathered by Gilovich, were dismissed as the work of a crank. Logic and proof could not possibly outweigh their experience and intuition. And the belief lives on today.

Why do we detect patterns that are not there, and why do we insist they are real? Social scientists think that early human beings survived by evolving an ability to detect patterns in nature. Observing the coming and going of herds of animals allowed the primitive hunter to kill more efficiently, assuring the survival of the tribe. And since so much depended on these newly recognized patterns, humans learned to take them quite seriously. The problem is that we have now become so efficient at the detection of patterns that we often see them when they are not there at all. Just as I "discovered" the sequence of taps that would ring the bell in the museum, we have become expert in knowing what isn't so.

And so we see our modern examples. It is easy to imagine that the birth of a baby born when the moon is full will be remembered more easily than other births, and it won't take many such memories to irrevocably cement our belief that more babies are born on lunar nights. A long run of successful basketball shots will be linked in our minds to that first basket, and no power on earth can convince us that hands do not become hot. We cannot escape the fondness our minds have for the detection of patterns.

When we make our medical decisions we must not fall into the same trap. We must realize how easy it is to see patterns that are not there. Such treachery arises when we want to evaluate a new medical treatment. Does the treatment really cure the disease? Or are we being fooled by false patterns as the disease naturally appears and disappears, only seemingly affected by the treatment?

This question is at the heart of medicine, since the basic task of medicine is to provide treatment that really works. We have been fooled in the past, as in the era of bloodletting and clysters, and we are being fooled now as millions waste their money and health on quack remedies. Our charge to ourselves is to ignore those patterns that just aren't so.

Patterns are your friend. Patterns are your enemy.

Coincidence *versus* the Scientific Method

My wife and I have a running argument about treatment of the common cold, an argument that neither of us will ever win. She claims that if I would just take a Super-Mega-Multivitamin every day, my cold symptoms will vanish within one week. I can't resist arguing that since most cold symptoms vanish in about a week anyway, the treatment with vitamins or whatever is completely superfluous and probably useless. She then counters with a story of a friend who didn't take vitamins and went on to have a cold for months (more about testimonials later), and besides, how did I know that the cold wouldn't have lasted even longer without the vitamins?

From my wife's point of view, the utility of these medications is a proven fact. Over and over again, she has used the medications and her cold has always gone away. From my point of view, this is the trap that

Gilovich warned us about. We notice that our cold goes away after we use the medication, but it would have vanished anyway. You might as well say that we have proven that taking the medication causes the sun to rise the next morning. (Powerful vitamins, indeed, I snicker.)

At times when my courage is high, I have told my wife that her way of reasoning also proves that drinking milk causes cancer, since almost everyone who has ever had cancer has had a glass of milk sometime in their lifetime. And there is always the argument that the wind is caused by trees moving. But I am rarely that brave....

So who is right, and how do we tell? Clearly, no amount of further sophistry or bickering will convince either side. What I would like to ask you now is to close this book and think for a few moments how you would solve this before reading on. I'll wait for you in the next paragraph....

What did you come up with? Perhaps something like this: Let's take two comparable groups of people with colds, and give vitamins to just one of the groups. If the groups recover from their colds in an equal amount of time, then we can say vitamins don't work. If the vitamin group recovers earlier, then my wife is right, and I will have to begin taking my vitamins.

Chances are that whatever you came up with, it represents the scientific method. Far from an abstract principle or a sinister intellectual concept, the scientific method is just a particular set of ways to test cause-and-effect relationships in a very, very skeptical fashion. Its goal is to prevent our falling into traps like those described by Gilovich.

A more chilling example is that of the drug laetrile, a medication derived from kernels of stone fruits such as apricots, once thought to be effective in treating cancer. The proponents of this drug noticed that some patients who took laetrile did well for a relatively long period of time. What they did not consider was that some patients do well without laetrile, and that other patients taking laetrile do poorly. When these considerations were taken into account, scientists found that not only was laetrile of no benefit, but that its use could be harmful. An incomplete analysis of data can be dangerous.

We have seen that the power that data has over us is no accident, for human beings have survived over the eons by noticing the patterns of nature around them, reacting to all sorts of fantastic theories of cause and effect. These qualities enabled us to avoid predators, take timely shelter from storms, and ultimately create great civilizations. But these forces also gave the human mind the dubious skill of seeing patterns that aren't really there. Nobel Prize-winning immunologist Sir Peter Medawar summed it up for the case of medicine: If a man recovers from an illness after a treatment, then "no power of reasoning known to medical science can convince him that it may not have been the treatment that restored him to health."

We are easily fooled by the complexity of nature and by our own minds. And the stakes are high. We must therefore always be prepared for a struggle when we attempt to distinguish medical reality from mere patterns.

Cause and effect are treacherous in medicine.

BELIEFS BASED ON SMALL NUMBERS

Let me illustrate a common problem of medical research by describing an experiment that will seem a bit odd.

Suppose you are in Las Vegas, and you want to study which numbers are obtainable by rolling dice. You take one of a pair, roll it and get a 1. You repeat this, getting a 3, and repeat it once more, this time again getting a 1. You then conclude that the only numbers obtainable from throwing a single die are 1 and 3, with 1 occurring twice as often as 3.

If you believed these results, you would lose your shirt at the betting tables, of course, since your next roll is as likely to yield a 2 or a 5 as it is to yield a 1 or a 3. But what is wrong with our scientific experiment? We had a hypothesis (only certain numbers are obtainable), we took some data (rolled the die), and we summarized the results. Isn't that what scientists do?

The answer, of course, is that we did not gather enough data. We all know that with more trials, we would obtain all the other numbers between 1 and 6. The exact number of throws we need to settle the issue may not be completely obvious, but it is clear that we need many more than three in order to ascertain the outcomes of rolling dice.

Now look what happens in medical research. Suppose you are reading a study of a new drug for breast cancer. You read that the study contains two groups of women; the first group was given a standard drug, and the second group was given the new drug. So far so good. But now you begin to realize just how complex matters can become. The women will be of different ages, and may have different stages of breast cancer, or even different types. Some may have already received chemotherapy or radiation, and some may not. Some of the tumors will be more aggressive than others. Some of the women may elect to leave the study before its end, some may die. There may be a wide variation in reporting of symptoms, and tumors may progress after the study ends.

You then read that there will be fifteen women in each group. Do you believe the conclusions of the study? Probably not. If it takes twenty or thirty or more throws just to determine the behavior of something as simple as dice, it is hard to believe that a study based on only fifteen women in each group will reflect what is really going on for something as complex as breast cancer. You just need more data.

But what if the study showed that the drug really seemed to work, so that ten of the fifteen women receiving the new drug had great results. Even with small numbers, you might be tempted to believe the study in this case. But beware. These great results could have happened by random chance, and if you repeated the study on the next fifteen women you might find dismal results. Statisticians call this a *regression to the mean*, but the bottom line is that small numbers can be frightfully deceptive.

The good news is that most scientists are aware of this problem, and that most will use well-accepted statistical tests to determine how many patients need to be included to produce valid conclusions. You may read that the results of the study were "significant," or that the study had adequate "statistical power," both terms indicating that these tests were used and that the numbers were large enough to support the conclusions. We learned about the concept of significance earlier. (See also the Recommended Reading list on page 259 for further information.) And this should make you more confident that the conclusions put forth are valid.

But don't relax completely. Statistical tests sometimes fail and are sometimes used incorrectly. Maintain your vigilance if the study you are reading uses small numbers of patients. The results may be valid, or may lead you to further useful reading, but they have to be taken with a very skeptical grain of salt.

Small numbers have small significance.

BELIEFS BASED ON BAD CHOICES: SELECTION BIAS

There is yet another major trap waiting for us in the medical literature.

A recent publication in the neurosurgical literature studied patients with a particularly aggressive type of brain tumor. This article reported that the patients who had most of their tumor surgically removed went on to survive longer than those who did not. The conclusion was that patients with these types of tumors should undergo aggressive surgery.

Who could doubt this? It certainly seems reasonable that removing more tumor should be of more benefit. And there is no doubt that the survival rates in this study were better when the tumors were aggressively removed. But there is a subtle problem in our way. This problem is called *selection bias*.

The problem lies in how these patients were chosen for surgery. Ideally, half of the patients would be randomly chosen to receive surgery, without regard for the state of their health or the size of their tumor. Instead, patients receiving surgery were chosen because their doctors believed they would do well with surgical procedure. Perhaps their tumors were small, near the brain's surface, or in nonessential parts of the brain, making removal a safer and easier task. Patients with larger tumors—those who were at a higher risk, surgery or not—were not chosen for an operation. It is no wonder, then, that the group receiving maximum removal did better. Their good results had more to do with the nature of their tumor to begin with than the amount of tumor that was removed. Even more disturbingly, if we believe the study enough to advise aggressive surgery to all patients with these tumors, we will seriously injure those who would not have been chosen for surgery; after all, they were not chosen because their tumor size or location was unfavorable. We would hurt more than help.

Experiments that divide patients into equally matched groups without bias are called *randomized trials*. They are considered by scientists to be the gold standard of research, the most believable of all scientific efforts. In fact, many doctors will not accept any medical assertion that has not been proved by such a trial, no matter how intuitively appealing.

Randomized trials, however, are difficult to perform. They deny the new treatment to the "control" group of patients, and usually require the expense and time it takes to collect years of data. Not every medical question has been studied with a randomized trial, and not every question will be so studied in the future. Imagine explaining the scientific benefits of withholding surgery to a patient with a fractured arm or an easily removed colon tumor.

So beware. As you read medical articles, you will find randomized trials mixed together with less scientific descriptions of clinical results. The randomized trials are more believable but also relatively scarce, while the more common descriptions are plagued by bias. Cherish the trials when you see them, but don't fail to appreciate the descriptions. They are often all we've got.

Randomization is the gold standard.

Beliefs Based on Single Reports

If you are an extreme coffee-drinker like myself, you would have been as interested and alarmed as I was several years ago when I ran across an article showing that drinking coffee causes pancreatic cancer. Never mind that pancreatic cancer is one of the most dreaded and deadly of tumors. The mere suggestion that my beloved habit might lead to any problem at all was disturbing enough to ruin my morning ritual with coffee and newspaper. The worst part about the article was that everything seemed to be in order: reputable scientists, a good journal, a randomized study, all the statistics in place. Should I have then given up caffeine for good? Would you?

The answer is no, not until someone else comes up with the same results. Scientists call this demand *reproducibility*, and it means that we should not believe anything that has been proven only once. The reason is that real life is just too complex and unpredictable for any one study to have the final word. Anything can go wrong with a single study; patients can turn out to be atypical, batches of medications can go bad, subtle traps of thinking can plague the most sophisticated of scientists. The only insurance against the undetected unexpected is to see that the same results come from several different researchers at several different times.

A good example was seen when Martin Fleischmann and Stanley Pons announced in 1989 that they had achieved cold fusion in their laboratory at the University of Utah. The news media were frantic, since this technical advance would have provided a new power source for the entire world that would have disrupted many aspects of the political and economic status quo. The immediate response of the scientific community was to try to replicate their work. It's not that other scientists thought that Fleischmann and Pons were liars or incompetent; that's just how science is. And when their results could not be replicated by other laboratories, it was clear that in fact, cold fusion was not yet a reality.

So when you read about how well a new drug works for angina, or when you see on the Internet that a new operation works better than the old one, or when the newspaper reports yet another breakthrough in treating disease with gene therapy, don't believe it unless it's been done more than once. Remember it, file it in your memory for later use, and seek out more information, but you cannot trust a result that has only been proven a single time. Once is not enough.

And for those of you who are worried, the article about coffee and pancreatic cancer was found to have a subtle but fatal statistical flaw. Our coffee time, at least for now, remains safe.

Once is not enough.

THE NEED FOR A GUIDE

Throughout the course of this book I have been strongly encouraging you to read about your medical problem. Read medical books, articles of all types, use the Internet, and use the tools I described earlier. You can never read too much. As one mentor once told me, the art is long, and life is short. . . .

But it is important to know your limits, too. The medical literature on any one topic is vast, contentious, and conflicting. For any medical disagreement, there are dozens of papers on each opposing side of the argument. Some of the papers are outdated quickly, some fall into the traps mentioned in the last two chapters, some are colored by commercial interests, and some are misleading. Don't be fooled by the calm, scientific phrases or the modern typesetting: The world of medical literature is a harsh and treacherous jungle. You need a guide.

That goes for me, too. I recently needed to know something about the treatment of a tumor called a sarcoma. This is a malignant tumor arising in soft tissues (the forearm, for example), but is rarely found in the brain. Although I am accustomed to reading the medical literature for neurosurgery, it was difficult for me to discern what was really true and what was more likely opinion from the articles that I read. I needed a guide, and I turned to my colleagues who were sarcoma experts for advice.

Unless you are an expert in your own medical problem, you need a guide, too. There is simply too much out there in too much disarray to easily make sense of it all. But does that mean you should stop reading and simply do what your doctor says? Absolutely not. Reading will teach you the tradeoffs and the difficulties inherent to your problem, and may suggest avenues of treatment to your doctor that he or she otherwise would not have considered. I am strongly suggesting, however, that you use your doctors to gain a sense of which ideas are good ones, which are dubious, and which are foolish. You don't have to agree in the end, and you can choose your own beliefs, but your doctors can be invaluable guides through the jungle.

You need both a guide and a guidebook.

BELIEFS ABOUT TESTIMONIALS

I hope this section will provoke you a bit, for I intend to attack one of our most trusted sources of information: the testimonial.

All of us are routinely and profoundly swayed by other people. We may have a friend who urges us to shop at his grocery store because he thinks the seafood is wonderful there, or a brother who insists we use the medicine that he says cured him of a recent illness. Our reliance upon testimonials is to be expected, since these are the stories that tell us about the world. From primitive times forward we have enjoyed stories, stories that contain valuable information of immense benefit. One might even suspect that our minds are built to receive information in the form of stories. As children we delight in fairy tales, and as adults we flock to the cinema. We receive our nightly news in the form of a story told through television. Testimonials give us vivid images that stick in our minds like no other data can.

Testimonials are not just enjoyable; they are essential to our daily lives. After all, no one person can gather firsthand experience about every aspect of existence. We depend on the testimonials of others to keep us well informed and knowledgeable.

But not all stories and testimonials are trustworthy. Advertisements, of course, are not widely trusted. Who really believes the woman on television when she assures us that her brand of detergent is really the best? Some of my favorite testimonials are those of gamblers who have written books, claiming to teach you how to win big in Las Vegas. If they really knew how to do this, would they be writing books?

Nor are well-meaning testimonials always true. The firsthand medical experience reported to you by your most trusted friend might be completely different from what will happen to you. Or your friends might be mistaken or careless about their information. You can't completely trust the friendly voices, either.

Testimonials are not just what your neighbor tells you. Testimonials are found everywhere, alive and well in our modern minds. I recently watched a popular talk show in which a "posture therapist" was demonstrating his craft. The therapist had studied a young woman the day before who suffered from migraine, and was now telling us that her headaches were caused by a hip asymmetry that put most of her weight on her right foot. And sure enough, to the delight of the audience, she was leaning on her right foot even as the therapist spoke. Relating migraine to posture is a bit of a conceptual reach, so that the talk show host turned to the therapist, and asked, "Does this really work?" With a look of sincerity, the therapist squared his body and said emphatically, "Beyond a shadow of a doubt."

And that settled that.

Claims like this make me angry. Perhaps posture therapy might help some patients with migraine, but you'll have to prove it to me with some form of a responsible study. You wouldn't buy a car based on a single unsupported assertion; why should you be less careful about your health?

Even if we know that testimonials are treacherous, they remain powerful sources of persuasion. Imagine, for example, what you would think if three of your closest friends developed serious liver failure after taking a particular antibiotic. Would you also take that antibiotic? What if you read several excellent scientific studies reporting that the chances of this drug causing liver failure were less than 0.001%? Would you believe the studies or would you heed the experiences of your friends? It is clear that even the most objective and rigorous scientific studies can be derailed by a small handful of testimonials.

I promised to provoke you, so here goes. As far as testimonials go, you can't trust advertisements; you can't trust television; you can't trust your enemies; you can't even trust your friends or family. Testimonials are stories about what happened to an individual; even if that individual loves and cares for you, you cannot assume that their story will happen to you.

Testimonials do have their uses, however, even if we do not believe them at face value. If your friend Michael did well after a type of surgery that you are considering for yourself, it might be wise to check it out, read about that operation, and ask your doctor. If Aunt Bea swears by Dr. X., it would make sense to investigate the reputation that Dr. X. may enjoy, good or bad, among other patients and doctors. And if you read that a particular drug worked in one patient, it would be good to find other articles about uses of the drug in groups of people and (of course) ask your doctor about it. Testimonials can be signposts, useful indicators to where the truth might be hiding.

Testimonials have another good use worth mentioning, and that is their ability to preserve hope. A 49-year-old woman with cancer might not be particularly thrilled to hear that the survival rate for people like her is only about 10% after five years. She would be delighted, however, to hear the details of a friend who survived more than twenty years with her type of cancer. Testimonials do provide proof that good events and outcomes are possible, and can be an uplifting beam of hope in otherwise dismal circumstances.

Beware of testimonials, especially those that seem real and bring tears to your eyes. For the best testimonials, the ones that affect us the most, are often the most deceptive. Testimonials are useful in guiding us to information that we might have otherwise overlooked, and they can be a source of hope. I am asking you to make a very difficult but crucial distinction between testimonials as proof of fact and testimonials as suggestions of what might, or might not, be true.

Beware the single story.

TEN

Step 6: Contemplation of Meaning

SUPPOSE YOU ARE FACED with a decision between two medical options, let's say between surgery and medication, to treat a liver condition. You do your homework and begin your analysis as I have advised. You identify your options and tradeoffs, then find and assess the available data, and then gather together your beliefs about medical matters. You would think at this point your task would be straightforward; simply pick the option that scored the best.

But in reality, it's not that easy. One more ingredient is missing. The surgery you are considering might have the best chance for cure, but the potential complications from infection might be so frightening that you choose medical treatment. Or one medicine for your psoriasis might clearly be the most effective, but you choose another since it is faster and you are tired of people staring. In the real world of medical decisions, there is rarely a single best decision; it is mostly a matter of meaning.

And so we must carefully consider the meaning of our decisions. We must identify which consequences are important to us, and discover why. We must develop practical strategies that will enhance our search for meaning. And we must acknowledge that this is a lonely quest, for meaning is an individual quality that cannot be obtained from others. But as elusive as the pursuit of meaning might seem, it is a pursuit commonly made and its ends commonly achieved. Here are some tips and perspectives that can help.

Meaning matters.

SLEEP ON IT!

The old adage is right. Don't be in a big hurry to make a decision. Go home and take your time. Sleep on it.

Admittedly, forcing yourself to delay your decision is not easy, especially when urgent medical issues are knocking at the door. We want our tumors treated yesterday, our heart attacks treated this moment. Nothing fuels anxiety more than a gap in the action.

The truth is, however, that except for true emergencies such as gunshot wounds, there is almost always time to take a step back, reflect on your choices, consult with others, and, yes, actually sleep on it. You wouldn't buy a car or a house on the spur of the moment; shouldn't you give yourself the same luxury when choosing your medical care?

Of course, sometimes time is of the essence. You would not want to take a month to decide how to treat a rapidly growing tumor, or take a week to finally begin that medicine for your irregular heartbeat. But in these cases, a single evening or even a few hours of reflection can lead you to better decisions and provide comfort about the options you have already chosen.

The problem we face is our modern attitudes about time. We are an action culture. We love fast-paced commercials and blitzkrieg movies, and we believe that every problem will yield to a "can do" attitude. We cope with our anxieties by "doing something" rather than by introspection. This is why surgery is such a seductive option; it is the ultimate form of "doing something" in response to a medical problem. To delay a dramatic intervention is frequently unbearable, not only for patients but also for their concerned physicians.

But this is the trap. Interventions and treatments may be dramatic, but that does not mean that they are what we really need. We should resist the temptation to act and resist being seduced by the fanfare of surgery or the spin of a new drug. One of the best ways to avoid this trap is to impose a small delay on your decisions. You will find that after a night's thought, the shine will fade and the true tradeoffs will emerge in your mind. Only then can you begin to approach a good decision.

So take your time. Don't make decisions in the doctor's office. Mull it over while you are in different moods, at different times of the day, and in different places. Talk with your family, friends, and consultants. Take long walks. Read. Dream. Sleep on it.

You'll be glad you did.

Resist the temptation to act.

THE ROAD TO MEANING

The great mathematician Henri Poincaré once told how he arrived at a particularly difficult mathematical insight that did not come from his usual careful and logical analysis. Instead, while boarding a bus during a tourist excursion, he noted that, "at the moment when I put my foot on the step, the idea came to me, without anything in my former thoughts seeming to have paved the way for it, [that] the transformations I had used to define the Fuchsian functions were identical with those of non-Euclidean geometry!"

Although this piece of subtle mathematics flashed unannounced into Poincaré's mind without any effort or direction, it is clear that he was familiar with the basic concepts. He knew all about Fuchsian functions, and I suspect he had thought about them for long hours. It was this intense thinking that prepared his mind for his later unexpected vision.

And so it is with medical decisions. Just because you've decided to sleep on a decision does not mean you should sleep through it. Your thoughts need to rummage through the attic of your mind, examining now this bit of information and now that, percolating to a decision behind the scenes of your conscious activity. Like Poincaré, you must actively decorate your mental attic, supplying your unconscious mind with the raw materials it needs in the labor of its decision. It is not enough to relax and allow your mind to magically act; you must first do the hard work of seeking medical information and of ruminating and reflecting on its meaning before the insights will burst into your conscious mind. And burst they will, at times and places you least suspect, seemingly out of nowhere.

Reflecting upon the facts while coming to a decision can be either pleasant or painful. One of my patients, Jeannie G., came to me seeking advice on what to do about a rare malformation of blood vessels embedded in her brain. She had heard vaguely about surgery and about radiation therapy, but her efforts to decide on a course of action were frustrated by what appeared to me to be circular thinking. When I gave her some basic information about these treatments—descriptions, efficacy rates, risks, pros and cons—she visibly relaxed over the course of just a few minutes. It was not that she had made a specific decision or chosen a plan of action. Rather, it was as if she instinctively knew that the facts were laid open for her and that her mind was prepared for the next stage of subconscious rumination that would lead to a good and comfortable decision.

Remember to give your subconscious the time it needs to sift through all the data. Don't jump to a decision early in your thinking process; let your mind float above it all, avoiding early commitments to any particular plan of action. Keep your mind open. This is not easy, since the gravity of your medical needs will pull you earthward toward the comfort of a quick decision. But floating like this for a while lets you take stock of the big picture and will ultimately result in better choices.

Decisions come to a prepared mind.

USE YOUR IMAGINATION

How do you shop for clothes? Do you select something at random from the clothes rack and wait until you are home before you try it on? Of course not. You try on the best candidates in the store, before you buy anything, rejecting the ones that don't fit and taking the one that feels and looks the best.

We can do the same to explore the meanings of the different possibilities lying within our medical decisions. Although we can't "try on" each medical possibility like we try on a coat, we can try each possibility by making use of our imagination. By experiencing the different consequences of our decisions in our mind's eye, we can discover meanings that we would otherwise not notice.

Here is one simple technique to get started. Set aside some time for yourself, alone from others and preferably in a quiet place. Close your eyes, or gaze into the distance, and list to yourself the different options you are facing. Your list may be short—for example, surgery and chemotherapy—or it may be a list of drugs, or a list of surgeries. Then, for each option, imagine all the outcomes, good or bad, that might happen. For surgeries, list the complications, for drugs, list the side effects, and so on. Make a special effort to include all the bad events that could possibly happen.

Now, to yourself what it would be like to live with each of these choices. Take your time here, and be as detailed as you can. If the surgery you are contemplating to remove a tumor might result in a paralyzed leg, try to imagine what it would be like to wake up in the morning with a leg that does not work. How will you get around? Will you need help? How will your family respond? How will you cope at the workplace, and how will you manage with daily chores? Imagine the opposite as well; imagine not having the surgery. How will you do with the alternative of chemotherapy? How frightening will your life be without the security of tumor removal? How will you cope with tumor spread that could interfere with breathing? Will you blame yourself if the tumor progresses to paralyze your leg anyway? How will your family respond in that case?

It is important to be as detailed as you can be, to try to imagine what it would really be like to live with each situation. And it is important to include as many of the unpleasant possibilities as you can. Don't be concerned with how rare each situation might be. You just want a taste of each option. You can consider the odds of each occurrence later.

Be prepared to cry. You are imagining the unthinkable, the destruction of the integrity of your body and of your life. You are visualizing what most people cannot ever let themselves see. There may even be times when this exercise may be so painful that you have to stop (and that's okay).

This exercise is difficult for another reason: Most people are not very good at predicting their future feelings. Two scientific studies cited by epidemiologist and physician Redelmeier show just how bad we are at this task. One study showed that people could not accurately predict whether they would continue to like a certain flavor of ice cream if they ate it every day for a week. A second study (we mentioned this one earlier) compared the quality-of-life ratings of two groups. One group consisted of people who had won the lottery the year before, the other was composed of accident victims who had been paraplegic for one year. It's hard to believe, but these groups rated the quality of their lives identically. Our predictions of how we will manage in the future are frequently wrong.

However uncertain and painful, the exercise of imagery can be invaluable in finding the personal meanings of your medical options. And these meanings may be surprising. You may find that loss of a leg is not as devastating as you first thought, or that the addition of an injected medicine to your schedule is simply intolerable. Again, no right answers, just individual insights from your personal explorations.

Try it on for size.

REPEAT IT OVER AND OVER

We are not computers, able to arrive instantly at a result in one fell swoop without rehearsal and rumination. Instead, we require a certain amount of repetition of our thoughts as we struggle with difficult decisions. We may find that we rehearse our arguments as we drift off to sleep, or repeat our thoughts to tedium as we discuss our decisions with others. To be sure, endless repetition without resolution is to be avoided. But let yourself repeat, and rehash, and restate, and rehearse, for that is how the human mind turns over a problem to its resolution.

Play it again and again.

KEEP NOTES

What did Samuel Pepys, Charles Darwin, and Leonardo da Vinci have in common? At least one thing: They all kept notes. These great men knew that writing down one's thoughts not only helps retrieve them later, but also promotes the clarity of mind leading to completely new insights. And so they wrote, regularly and copiously, to themselves and to the world.

This is no less true for medical matters, and no less helpful for our medical decisions. I strongly recommend that you keep a personal journal of your thoughts and feelings as you make your medical decisions. You don't have to produce a finished piece of literary art; just jot down a few short phrases describing your thoughts as they occur. Write down your impressions of your choices when you first learn about them, then again after you have done some reading, then again after discussions with your doctors. Write honestly and write to yourself, giving it the flavor of a diary.

You may recall I advised you to keep a diary of the strategic details of your medical journey. I asked you to record which doctor said what, the results of lab tests, and the myriad details of medical appointments that are so quickly forgotten. Now I am advising you to write something different: a record of your subjective thoughts and feelings. It may be convenient to keep these two journals together, but remember that they are two distinct works.

The very act of writing will crystallize your thoughts and prepare your mind to receive new ideas. Reviewing your journal will not only be personally interesting, but will give you insight into what is meaningful for you and will suggest future directions. Whether you enjoy writing or consider it a chore, keeping a record of your subjective meanings is priceless.

Write it down.

THE MEANING OF RISK

In his insightful book, *The Psychology of Judgment and Decision Making*, Scott Plous gives the following example, which he attributes to economist Zeckhauser. Suppose you were playing Russian roulette and you knew there was only a single bullet left in your revolver. How much would you pay to remove this one bullet before your next turn?

Now suppose that you knew that there were four bullets in your revolver. How much would you pay to remove just one of them?

Most people would pay more to remove the single bullet than one of the four bullets, feeling that the perfect safety of no bullets at all was worth more than the relative safety of fewer bullets. And in fact, a variety of studies have shown that people in general would much rather eliminate risk than merely reduce it. When we apply this to medical choices, we have to ask: How much are we willing to sacrifice for perfect safety?

You may recall that we discussed the interpretation of small risks earlier in this book. I cautioned you that we could never eliminate all risk or ensure perfect safety. All we can do is compare our estimates of risks with commonplace events, so as not to worry unduly about levels of risk that we normally accept in our everyday life. Now we must go further; we must consider the meaning of what we must do to reduce risk.

Suppose, for example, that a certain surgery to remove your malignant tumor had a success rate of 95%, but also had an 8% chance of complications that would result in leg paralysis. How far would you go to lessen or eliminate the chance of complications? Would you accept an 80% success rate if the complication rate could be reduced to 5%? Or a 50% success rate if the complications could be reduced to 2%? What about a 30% success rate for a complication rate of zero? There is no right answer, of course. It is more a matter of style.

As suggested by this example, we can fall into the trap of diminishing returns, in which we begin trading more and more success for reductions in risk that are so small as to be meaningless. But just exactly what "meaningless" should be is up to you, and this threshold will be different for different people. You must decide at what point the added expense is worth a reduction in risk, based on what the risky consequences mean to you.

Only you can decide when better is the enemy of good enough.

THE MEANING OF DETAILS

Linda D. is a petite, soft-spoken 28-year-old woman with long, auburn hair who has had epilepsy for most of her life. Her seizures now occur about twice a week and have continued without warning despite many attempts to control them with medications. During her seizures, she babbles and gags and screams, then shakes her right side as if thrashed by a demon, then shakes all over and loses consciousness. Occasionally she urinates on herself or bites her tongue. People around her become frightened, even if they already know she has seizures. Understandably, she has been unable to hold a job and is worried that she will become a burden to her family. She tries to maintain a positive attitude, but a growing difficulty with depression is beginning to get the best of her.

Highly motivated to improve her circumstances, Linda has spent two years being formally evaluated by the epilepsy group at our hospital. This evaluation includes in-depth neurologic testing, MRI scans, EEG recordings, SPECT scans, and psychological, cognitive, and social evaluations. The purpose of this intricate protocol is to determine whether Linda's seizures come from a part of her brain called the temporal lobe, and whether surgical removal of that part might alleviate her seizures. Fortunately for Linda, the tests showed that surgery would indeed have a high probability of success.

And so Linda and her family came to me to discuss this operation. I described the details of the surgery for Linda and her family, as well as the potential complications. They listened quietly and attentively, asking a few questions along the way, seeming to understand all the information. Included in the discussion were the more serious complications of death and paralysis that only rarely occur.

Toward the end of this discussion, Linda spoke up and asked, "Will you have to shave my hair?" I answered yes, but that this could be limited to a narrow strip of hair along the incision. And in any case, her hair would grow back.

She looked down at the floor, shaking her head to herself in a way that allowed her hair to hide her face. "No way," she said. " I'm not going to do this if you shave my hair." Then she was silent.

After a pause, her mother leaned forward, trying without success to look in her eyes, and said softly, "But Linda honey, your hair will grow right back. The doctor has to shave a little to do the operation."

"I don't care," Linda replied, determined but not angry, and still looking at the floor. "I'm not going to do this if they have to shave my hair."

And so ensued a quiet, intense discussion between Linda and members of her family about whether she should forgo the surgery for which she had prepared for years just to avoid having her hair shaved. As I listened to Linda defending her wishes to her family, I thought that perhaps the action of shaving had become a symbol to Linda for the serious complications so calmly accepted a few minutes before. Reopening the discussion again to these complications was the key; Linda ultimately agreed to the surgery and happily had no further seizures.

Like Linda, all of us have issues that outwardly do not make much sense to others but have great symbolic significance to ourselves. To Linda, shaving her hair stood for the lack of control and the frightening risks attached to her surgical operation. For many people, the tedium of waiting for the doctor, the pain of the needle used to take blood, the humiliation of an insurance interview, or any of the thousands of annoying details in the experience of being a patient can trigger strong feelings of anger and resentment that often disguise fear and apprehension.

These sensitivities are normal, hiding deep within our mental forests. Our friends and families will not understand their significance, and may become angry and frustrated with us. They may lose patience, withdrawing emotional support when we need it most. And sadly enough, not all physicians will recognize these symbols as subtle clues to more substantial worries. They may dismiss you as noncompliant or belligerent. We ourselves, therefore, must recognize the validity of our worries that seem small and irrational, and understand their meaning; they are normal ways in which we experience the fear and anxiety arising from being ill. We can then turn our full attention to the important issues and let the unimportant details remain unimportant.

Minor worries hide major fears.

THE MEANING OF INCONVENIENCE

Georgia M. is a plump, matronly 72-year-old woman who came to my office to discuss treatment of her recently found tumor. I explained some facts to her about her problem and discussed some of her options. I began listing some of the risks of treatment, including stroke and death, so that she could begin to mull over her choices. But as soon as I uttered these words, her eyes widened and she sighed, "Oh my God. Death?"

I replied yes, but assured her that the risk of death was low. I then described one of the treatments that would require that she be in Dallas several times over the next few weeks. She looked at me as if I had slapped her in the face. "But I live a hundred and twenty miles away. How am I going to get here?"

I really didn't want to shock her any further with unpleasant details, but I had to go on. She would have to have routine MRI scans yearly, probably forever ("Oh my God, forever? I can't do that!"). I could not guarantee that insurance would pay for all of her expenses ("What am I going to do?"). And there was a chance that she would require certain medications for a long time ("I really don't like to take medicine. Are you sure?").

Just when I was certain that my speech had wounded her beyond any hope of repair, she leaned forward, looked me straight in the eye, and calmly said, "All those things don't matter. The only thing I want you to do is take care of my tumor. I don't want to die. I'll figure out how to deal with all that stuff. You just get me the right treatment."

I was touched and impressed by her transformation. A moment ago, she was obsessed with the inconveniences of being a patient. Now she was dead serious about beating her tumor. And her seriousness was contagious, cementing my commitment to do everything I could to help her fight her disease.

We've seen how small details can stand for fear and anxiety. In a similar fashion, the inconveniences of being a patient often take on their own meaning. They can dominate our thinking, swaying us towards the wrong decisions. We may decide that it is not worth the extra thirty minutes in the car to see a skilled expert, or that we cannot miss an extra day of work to undergo a better type of treatment. Sometimes our medical problems are indeed so minor that it really is not worth enduring any extra inconvenience. But even seemingly minor medical problems can have serious consequences that will be with us forever. Most often, better care is worth the inconvenience.

Let inconvenience rule.

THE MEANING OF THE PAST

Chances are, you are no stranger to medical decisions, and I'm willing to bet that you have made many in the past. Perhaps most of your decisions have been relatively minor, although most people have faced at least one major medical decision by the time they reach adulthood. But in either case, it is worth reflecting on whether your past decisions were good or bad, and what made them that way. The past has much to teach.

For example, if you chose a surgical treatment instead of taking medicines, was the outcome what you expected? Was the recovery time tolerable? Did the "minor problems" associated with surgery, such as numbness or change in body image, have a major effect upon you? Or did you even notice them?

As another example, if you chose to monitor your blood glucose or cholesterol rather than treating it more aggressively with medication, were you happy in the long term? Do you find watching your lab values to be nerve-wracking, and find yourself wishing for definitive therapy? Or is the process of watching comforting to you, since you know it frees you from the complications of the medicines you chose not to take?

If you now face a medical problem similar to one you faced in the past, your decision may be especially difficult. For example, suppose you elected to have a tumor treated with radiation rather than surgery twenty years ago, knowing that radiation leads to a cure rate of 90%. Now you find that the tumor has nevertheless recurred, so you are again faced with the choice of radiation or surgery. Would you choose radiation again, relying again on its high rate of cure? Or would you choose surgery, based on your unusual and unlucky experience with radiation?

Each of our medical problems is unique, of course, and what we did in the past is not always the correct answer for the present. And unless your medical problem is stubbornly recurrent, the particulars will be different every time you face a medical decision. But remembering how your decisions turned out in the past can often guide you to insight that will make you happy in the future.

Let experience be your teacher.

THE MEANING OF STYLE

How did you choose the color of your car? Why did you choose a sporty red or an elegant white? How about your clothes—do you wear old jeans or more fashionable slacks? What about your music, your hair length, your watch? What goes into those choices?

A major ingredient in any of our choices is style. Dictionaries tell us the word *style* comes from the Latin *stilus*, denoting the pointed stick used for writing long ago. And although *style* was first used to describe the manner in which we used these sticks to express ourselves in writing, it now characterizes the multitude of ways we express ourselves in the thousands of details of our lives. Though intangible, style is a powerful force behind each of our decisions.

And it would be naive to believe that medical decisions are immune from the influence of our personal style. True, the making of a medical decision is a serious business that can determine life or death. But these decisions come from us, from our desires and preferences and experiences, and can no more be unaffected by our individual style than can our choice of clothing in the morning.

Nathan K. is a surgeon with a problem. The vision in his left eye has been worsening for many years, and it is now so poor that he can barely make out newspaper headlines. But his surgical ability has not suffered because his right eye is still good and he has quietly learned to adapt during the slow decline of his left. He knows that an operation could dramatically improve his vision, but the risk of losing his left eye altogether is not small and could end his career. Yet, his left eye is worse each month.

How will Nathan make his decision? He will look into the facts, the risks of surgery, the possible outcomes. As we discussed in the last section, he will undoubtedly be swayed by his beliefs—his belief in the virtues (or evils) of surgery, for example. And he will contemplate the personal meaning that each possible outcome has for him.

But he will also be moved by his personal style. Like many surgeons, he may live for action, and the thought of feeling his eye slowly deteriorate may be intolerable when he could *do* something, when he could have the operation. Or he may be the cautious type (as many surgeons are), willing to let it be until absolutely necessary.

Be aware of your style, and be glad for it. It will guide you through tough decisions, and make understandable those decisions that might otherwise seem arbitrary. And an appreciation of your style will help you find decisions that are tailored for you, not for someone else.

Don't discount style.

THINKING THE UNTHINKABLE

Have you ever been so scared of something that you could not bring yourself to look at it?

I hope not, but for those of you who have had cancer, or a heart attack, or any other life-threatening event, I am willing to bet that this has happened to you. It seems obvious, but a key fact that escapes our families, friends, and many doctors is just how frightened we are when we are patients. It is one thing to sit in the doctor's office, calmly discussing medicines and options and schedules. It is quite another when we are alone with our thoughts at night. As patients facing major medical problems, we are terrified. And that is understandably normal.

It is also normal for this terror to become focused upon one or more objects or thoughts. You may be unable to look at your own chest X-ray, for example, or you may find yourself having difficulty finding the time to fill a particular prescription. It may be impossible for you to make plans in case something does go wrong, for contingencies such as the loss of a leg or a stroke. You may be unable to discuss your own death with your family even as plans are being made for that possibility.

This fact bears repeating: These difficulties are understandable and normal. But even so, despite the discomfort, you can learn to function and make good medical decisions. The first step is to be patient and give yourself some time for all the new and disturbing information to sink in and to be digested. You may find that what is unthinkable today is approachable in a week. Another tip is to allow yourself to be detached and intellectual about it all, at least temporarily. The only way that most people can plan for their own death, for example, is to push aside the natural feelings of fear and hopelessness with an intellectual focus on the details of the will and the funeral.

You may also find it helpful to sneak up on these issues, talking about the serious aspects of your problem a little bit more each day. And there are some things you don't need to do if you just don't want to; you probably don't need to look at your own chest X-ray as long as you can talk about what it means.

The important point is that you become able to process all the information one way or another. It is normal to have certain holes in your thinking surrounding the frightening aspects, but you should still be able to make plans and decisions, perhaps by intellectualizing or with a gradual approach. If certain aspects are so frightening that you cannot bring yourself to think about important issues and decisions, don't hesitate to seek professional help. This can be comforting, useful, and lifesaving. But usually an awareness that these are frightening times together with some care in navigating the frightening issues will be what you need to arrive at good decisions.

Fear is normal.

THE MEANING OF FAITH

"There are no atheists in foxholes."

In one short, pithy statement, the quotation above sums up what theologians and philosophers have taken volumes to say: Human beings are spiritual animals.

All of us have a spiritual side. Even the most stalwart atheist wonders about the universe, our place in it, and whether there is a purpose to what we see. And I think that having that sense of wonder counts as a spiritual side, even in the absence of more traditional beliefs.

At no other time is our spiritual side called forth more strongly than when we face a medical decision. For it is at this time that our way of life and our very existence are threatened. At these times we are fearful, perhaps more than at any other time in our lives. The questions of meaning, purpose, and comfort roll forward without effort from our struggle with illness.

Each of us will use our spirituality differently as we make our medical decisions. No general guidelines can be given, and no one solution can be said to be correct. But we can look at some examples. Some devout people believe in a benevolent God who will guide them to the correct decision. They have few conflicts about their decisions, and that is right for them. Others believe that God will help them with a decision only with prayer and rigorous ritual. This is the right way for them. I have had patients arrange their surgery to fall on dates dictated by astrology. This is the right thing for them. And some Jehovah's Witnesses, on the basis of their beliefs, would rather die than accept a blood transfusion. This is right for them.

Whatever your beliefs, don't neglect your spirituality. It is an important part of your thinking and will be present whenever you are threatened with a medical problem. Pay attention to that voice and let it guide you as you make your good medical decisions.

Spirituality matters.

Part III
How to Use Your Doctors

ELEVEN

Ambivalence, Anger, and Acceptance

BEFORE WE CAN FIND WAYS to best use our doctors, we must first understand something of our relationships with them. Although no one summary can fully portray the interaction of every patient with every doctor, two common themes, ambivalence and anger, seem to be universal. Let's examine the role each of them plays in our medical decisions.

AMBIVALENCE

We hate our doctors, and we love them too. We hate their power over us, their authority that reminds us we are ill and needy. But we love them for caring for us and for helping us escape the horrors of disease. We love them, we hate them; we are ambivalent.

The word *ambivalent* truly and accurately describes our feelings for doctors, since we attach such a great value (the *valent* part) to both (the *ambi* part) viewpoints. We want them to take care of us and make our decisions, but we also want to hold onto our autonomy and decide for ourselves. It is not that we are ambiguous, not knowing how we feel; we are truly ambivalent, vividly loving and hating doctors, personally and feverishly, both at the same time.

James K. is a good example. He is a 65-year-old rancher from Oklahoma who has been treated for a brain tumor for many years. Fortunately, his tumor is small and slow-growing and does not often require treatment. But when it does, his visit to my clinic is explosive.

As James stands in my office (he won't sit), you can see he is a tall man wearing a black Western-style shirt, a large metal belt buckle in the shape of a longhorn tucked beneath his ample belly, and yes, a cowboy hat and boots. My nurse tersely briefs me under her breath before I enter his room: he yelled at the receptionist, he insulted the nurses, he won't keep his other appointments. He is turning the clinic upside down.

But when I talk with him, he is all business, pleasantly talkative in a mellow country twang that is inviting and yet seems both overcultivated and subtly assertive. I have to admit he is a bit belligerent, but he and I are quickly able to agree on a plan that satisfies us both. He is not a problem.

James is the personification of ambivalence. On the one hand, he listens to my advice with military intensity and takes me as seriously as any general evaluating foreign intelligence. He needs this process of consultation and even seems to enjoy it. On the other hand, he hates being there, hates bending to the will of the clinic routine, and he won't even sit down.

We are all like James, although most of us are less obvious. We all harbor intense ambivalence, needing the doctor's help and empathy yet hating the unavoidable dependence. And we are all angry—sometimes furious—at having to relinquish our autonomy. How then, do we use our doctors to make good medical decisions when we are so distracted by our ambivalence and anger?

We love them, we hate them.

ANGER

Once again, we must accept that these so-called negative emotions—anger and resentment—are perfectly normal. Everyone feels at least a twinge of indignation when waiting for the doctor, and everyone has mixed feelings about being dependent even if their doctor is the most beloved of physicians.

But the trick is to not allow this anger to get in your way. Your goal is to make the best medical decisions possible, *not* to engage in a competitive struggle with your doctor. Be angry, accept the resentment springing from your temporary dependence, but put it aside and focus on the task at hand. Just as it is not fruitful to rage against the weather when it rains, so is it less than helpful to let your inevitable dependence on doctors affect your decisions. Be like James: ornery for sure, but focused on the issues of health.

Our ambivalence about doctors is so unsettling that it often leads to attempts to deny its existence altogether. An example is one of my pet peeves, the concept of "partnering" with your doctor. The idea is that the discomfort of our ambivalence for doctors will melt away if we can view them as an equal but differently endowed partner, an ally contributing just as much as we do to our medical care. But this doesn't work, any more than you can eliminate the discomfort of a hot sun on a summer's day by thinking of the sun as your partner in sustaining life. It's still hot and you still sweat. Denying the ambivalence won't make it go away; it is a normal and unavoidable part of the doctor-patient relationship.

The anger is normal.

Do We Really Want a Vote?

Some would argue that our ambivalence about doctors is irrelevant because in fact, most of us would rather let the doctor decide for us. Carl Schneider is an attorney and bioethicist who champions a provocative perspective in his book, *The Practice of Autonomy*. Based on his intensive studies of how people really make medical decisions, he believes that the modern, politically correct viewpoint—that people make decisions by subjecting carefully gathered medical information to an insightful, personal analysis—is wrong. Instead, he found that people harbor all degrees of ambivalence for the task of making medical decisions. Some want to decide everything for themselves, some want the doctor to decide everything for them, and many are somewhere in between. But more often than not, patients would like to say, "You're the doctor, you decide." And so perhaps we should abandon attempts at rational decision making, perhaps we should not waste precious time gathering and interpreting medical information, because in our hearts, that is not how we really want to make our medical decisions.

While no one would argue that medical decision making is ever completely rational, I do not think we should abandon attempts to gather medical data and think carefully about our medical decisions. Because in reality, we cannot. As human beings, we are simply unable to allow another to have absolute control of our decisions without some smoldering sense of discomfort. Even the patient who says "You decide" does not really mean "You decide everything, no matter what." Even these patients would rebel if the doctor chose a path leading to a lifetime of suffering or permanent separation from family. We all want some involvement in our fate, even if it is just a vote or a right to a veto.

And there is a practical matter. Our society will not tolerate giving complete decision authority to the doctor. We give too much lip service to personal autonomy, we are too suspicious of authority figures (political, medical, or otherwise), and the doctors won't take full responsibility for our decisions for fear of being sued. Even if we wanted our doctors to decide everything for us, it just won't happen.

So if you are not completely comfortable making your own decisions without the doctor, but you still want to be able to determine your medical fate, you are not alone. All of us want to give up some autonomy to the doctor, some more than others. But none of us wants to relinquish our right to vote.

Keep your power to vote.

ACCEPTANCE

So how do we pull our decisions together in the midst of these conflicting feelings about doctors and their care? How can we resolve our contradictory wishes to decide for ourselves and yet have the doctor decide for us?

The answer lies in understanding that the way we handle our ambivalence—the way we choose how much the doctor decides and how much we decide—is based largely on comfort, but that no decision can be perfectly comfortable. Some patients say they are most comfortable following their doctor's advice without question. But they cannot completely relax, since they must remain vigilant to veto decisions if they seem wrong. Others are more comfortable making their own decisions, but they cannot relax since they will be secretly listening to the doctor to make sure they have not chosen silly or dangerous options. The notion that we should follow our comfort might seem unsatisfactory to ethicists and might seem imperfect, since perfect comfort does not exist. But at a practical level, it is our sense of comfort that guides us through our difficult ambivalence, a sense unique for every person, based on an intangible inner compass poorly understood yet irresistibly powerful.

Comfort is king.

TWELVE

Managing Your Doctors

ALTHOUGH MUCH has been written about how to find a good doctor, most people rely on recommendations from friends or their own trusted physicians for referrals. It is beyond the scope of this book to detail this process further, but there are a few points to consider.

—FINDING DOCTORS—

DO I NEED A DOCTOR?

With all the medical information available at our fingertips, and with the sophistication of our modern computerized age, it may not seem worth the effort to obtain a doctor's advice. Why not just read about it on the Internet, ask a few friends, and make our own decisions?

My opinion? Yes, you need a doctor, especially for important medical issues. And consider this: Most people would be afraid to fix their car without the aid of a mechanic and most would be afraid to arrange their legal matters without an attorney. Is your medical care any less complex or important?

You need a doctor.

SECOND OPINIONS

I like the idea of second opinions. When facing tough decisions of any type, it makes a lot of sense to hear several viewpoints from several experts. In this way you will hear all the pros and cons, recognizing that no one expert can know it all.

Some patients are reluctant to ask for the names of other experts, for fear of angering or hurting the feelings of their own physicians. To them I would say: Good doctors do not mind requests for second opinions, and in fact welcome them. Doctors want their patients to be comfortable with their medical decisions, if for no other reason than to avoid malpractice lawsuits. And second opinions are excellent ways for patients to arrive at comfortable decisions.

Second opinions can also be difficult to obtain since they are expensive. Insurance companies frequently refuse to pay for a second opinion, and the expense of travel to another expert can be high. More than one patient has thought, "I really can't get a second opinion because the insurance company won't cover it."

In the case of a difficult decision, however, it may be worth the expense. Just because a second opinion is not covered by insurance does not mean that you are not allowed to pay for it yourself. You might also find that the cost of the consultation itself is not as high as you thought, although medical testing can become quite expensive. But an hour's time with an expert costs about the same as what we pay our car mechanic to look over a used car, and the advice you get may keep you from buying a lemon. The information and peace of mind may well be worth the money.

Second opinions are worth a second thought.

SMALL TOWN *VERSUS* BIG CENTER

Most people obtain their medical care close to home, from doctors they know well and from local hospitals. But medical options have become so complex that in many cases only the larger medical centers can offer the best of what is available. Complicated medical problems such as simultaneous pregnancy and leukemia are usually referred to these centers, but even common diseases such as cancer and heart attack may receive more innovative treatment in these specialized hospitals.

You may want to seek treatment at a specialized center, particularly if your medical problem is rare or if your medical progress is poor. You can also travel to these centers just to obtain a second opinion, with the hope that the treatment itself might be carried out at home. Keep in mind that the sophistication of these centers might very well be worth the expense.

Complex problems require complex care.

—Practical Tips for the Appointment—

"A physician uses various methods for the recovery of sick persons; and though all of them are disagreeable, his patients are never angry."
—Addison, quoted in *Samuel Johnson's Dictionary*

"God heals, and the doctor takes the fees."
—Benjamin Franklin

Our main contact with our doctors is through formal appointments, usually in their offices or exam rooms. The pressure to obtain information during these structured interviews can easily frustrate your efforts to gain useful information, and more than one patient has left the doctor's office without feeling informed or comforted. Here are a few tips that can help you use your time with the doctor in a way that leads to good medical decisions.

Bring a list of questions. It can be difficult to think on your feet in the bustle of the doctor's office, so write down your questions and concerns before you go. Ask your friends or family to help you, and let the list be as long as you like. Doctors are generally appreciative of your organization.

Bring your written materials. If you have found some impressive medical articles or Internet information, don't hesitate to bring them to your doctor. This is a good starting point for discussion and allows your doctor to address these sources directly. Be reasonable about how much you bring; reading a foot-high stack is a big demand!

Don't try to please your doctor. Some people find themselves minimizing their symptoms or fears in the doctor's office, feeling that they don't want to "bother" the doctor. Others are afraid that their questions about alternatives might anger the doctor, or that their concerns might be boring. They unconsciously feel a need to please the doctor.

Remember, the doctor is not your friend. He or she is not there to be entertained or to pass judgment upon you. Nor should you worry whether you have your doctor's approval. The doctor's task is to advise and help you through your medical problem, and the worst thing you can do is to withhold the information necessary for that responsibility. So give a full report, air all your fears, and let it all come out. Your doctor will be glad you did.

Ask tough questions. The more serious your medical problem, the tougher the questions you will have. Will I die? Will it hurt? How many of these operations have you done? How much do you charge? Are there other ways to treat this? Can you refer me to someone for a second opinion?

Don't be afraid of angering the doctor. The fact that these questions popped into your mind means that you need to hear them answered. It is your right, and even your duty to yourself, to ask them clearly. Most doctors will understand why you are asking and will answer honestly without taking offense. And if you encounter the rare doctor who becomes angry, you've learned something: find another doctor!

Beware of "what if it were you?" Once we learn that we face a difficult medical decision, we naturally want advice from our doctors. Questions such as "what would you do if it were you?" and "what if it were your mother?" are commonly asked as if to find out what the doctor really thinks.

But beware of these questions, because the answers you hear may lead you astray. For the fact is that your doctor is *not* you, and may not share all of your viewpoints and attitudes. It is like asking the waiter at a restaurant to bring you what *he* likes best; you may not like what you get.

Yet we all need guidance from our doctors beyond a bland explanation of medical options. It is fair to ask your doctor which options are most reasonable given your set of circumstances, and to ask why. But don't be too insistent to hear your doctor's personal preferences; this is one of those times when it really is all about you.

Recognize that your doctor may not be up to date. It is an unfortunate fact that no doctor is up to date on every medical issue; no one person, of course, can keep up with the overwhelming supply of new medical facts thrown at us by the thousands every day. Usually this is not a problem, and doctors generally strive to keep current. But on occasion you might find that your doctor does not seem to be informed on some important aspect of your medical problem. Perhaps he or she has not heard of a drug you read about, or doesn't know about a new type of surgery. When this happens, both patient and doctor are embarrassed and it can be unclear what to do.

Here you will have to use some common sense. It wouldn't be the end of the world if your doctor is unaware of an obscure article you found on the Internet—no one can know everything. But if he or she seems rusty on bigger issues—a new but publicized medication, for example—I would advise you to watch carefully what your doctor does. If your doctor accepts the new information in stride and plans to investigate further, you might choose to continue in his or her care. But if your doctor dismisses the information without a thought, or becomes defensive, you may choose to seek another opinion or change doctors altogether.

Help your doctor. It is critical that you provide your medical information to your doctor. He or she needs you to report your symptoms and medical problems as completely and accurately as you possibly can. Being organized helps, but don't worry about being elegant, since it is more important to tell all the facts clearly. Include what drugs you are taking, what surgery you've had, and other problems in the past. If your situation is complex, it might be a good idea to give your doctors a written list of your medications and a narrative of your medical history.

I have a family member who asked me for some medical advice after he had seen his doctor for several serious medical problems. When I asked what he had told his doctor, I was shocked to hear him say, "Nothing. He's the doctor; it's his job to figure out what's wrong with me." And then we argued for hours about whose job it is to do what. You know how family members are. . . .

Your doctor needs your help. Without it, he or she cannot discover your diagnosis and cannot formulate an intelligent plan of treatment. My family member discovered this the hard way, when his medical problems took a turn for the worse because he would not help his doctors. Don't let the same thing happen to you.

Plan your appointment.

—The Use of Doctors—

Since when do we *use* doctors?

In times past, we wouldn't think of *using* our doctors. To the contrary, we would give ourselves completely to their authority, following their instructions to the letter as obedient children heed their parents. There was no need to understand their reasons and even less desire to question their judgment, because we trusted them to take care of us. We wouldn't *use* them; we would *follow* them. They were *doctors*.

But no longer. We are beginning to view our doctors more as mechanics of the body than as benevolent healing authorities. In our search for technical medical care, we seem to be seeking a car mechanic for the flesh, a technician charged with the task of fixing our bodies rapidly, inexpensively, and under our careful direction. And just as we are reluctant to trust our car mechanics to carry out repairs without our supervision, we demand direct involvement in our medical care. We want to be kept informed about our bodies as well as our cars, and we want to choose the ways in which both will be repaired.

The problem is that no matter how strong our desire for a doctor-mechanic might be, we still need that one-to-one contact with a compassionate physician who has our best interests in mind, contact with an old-fashioned doctor who will protect us from disease and advise us about life's tough problems.

How then, do we best use doctors to help us arrive at our medical decisions? How do we make the mental transition from the kindly, parental doctor entrusted with our care to the modern medical mechanic under our supervision? And how do we blend these two icons so that we do not lose the better aspects of each?

The first step to answer these questions is to examine what doctors are, and what they are not.

We want to control both our car and our care.

USE YOUR DOCTOR AS A PROVIDER

There is not a doctor alive who is not furious at being called a "provider." The term "provider," a gift from insurance companies, tells us that medical care is a simple service with a simple set value. Calling a doctor "provider" sends the message that medical care can be practiced by recipe, giving us permission to ignore the crucial differences among patients that require unique consideration. A "provider" cannot feel the sacred trust between doctor and patient, a trust transcending economic concerns. The art of medicine is trivialized even more by the common practice of referring to anyone in the health profession as a "provider." In this accounting, all are equal: nurses, physical therapists, technologists, and physicians. No wonder doctors bristle when they receive a letter beginning with "Dear Provider."

But apart from accounting, the concept of the doctor as a provider is a good starting point for our new thoughts about medicine. For doctors have indeed become providers. Doctors no longer play the role of benevolent parents, making your decisions and giving instructions to be followed. Instead, doctors are now providers of information, advice, and care.

For example, suppose you go to your doctor, reporting that you have had some funny fluttering feelings in your chest that occasionally make you dizzy. After some questions and tests, your doctor tells you that you have an abnormality called an arrhythmia, an irregularity in your heartbeat which can be life threatening. He or she tells you that there are two different medicines for this condition. One works well, but might impair your thinking; the other leaves your head clear, but can fail to control the arrhythmia. Your doctor outlines the pros and cons of each, emphasizing the greater safety of the medication that might cloud your thinking. But then something interesting happens. Your doctor asks what *you* want to do. The decision of which medicine to take, or whether to be treated at all, has suddenly become yours.

Of course, doctors are often more directive and occasionally more parental than I have outlined here. And rightly so, since some medical decisions require specific action. There may only be one way to set a fracture or to treat certain types of blood pressure, and your doctor may feel that there are no other reasonable choices. Nevertheless, doctors nowadays are being less directive when several options are available. And most will quickly allow you to choose your own options if you ask.

Be aware of this as you consult with your physicians. If you expect to be told exactly what to do, you may be disappointed. But what you can expect is to be provided with all the crucial information, advice, and opinions that you need to make superb medical decisions.

Use what they provide.

Don't Use Your Doctor as a Friend

I have a relative who has spent a long time trying to decide whether to undergo a particular type of surgery. During a recent visit, we discussed his medical problems and options. Many of my sentences started with "If I were you, I would..." or "Here's what I would do..." and even "Just do this...." I was directive, as friends are, exhorting him to one course of action and then another as the conversation dictated.

But don't expect this from your doctor. A doctor's task is different from that of a friend, more weighty and less comforting. Advice from a friend given during the light banter of conversation can be easily ignored. But a doctor's explanation of your medical realities and advice about your serious choices are not so easily dismissed. So don't expect to be told "here's what I would do if I were you,"or "just do this." That kind of talk is for friends, not doctors.

Your doctor is not your friend.

DON'T USE YOURSELF AS A DOCTOR

If doctors are the final source of medical information and advice, why should we try to learn about our medical problems? Why not just listen to their explanations and follow their advice? Why even read this book?

The answer lies again in our analogy with auto mechanics, as I learned while in college. In those days, I tried to save expenses more than once by attempting to tune up my own car. I bought automotive books, special tools for valves, and devoted my weekends to the task. But to the great amusement of my friends, my efforts would always end with a tow to the nearest garage where the work could be done properly. I am simply not a car mechanic.

But this embarrassing experience was still valuable, even if I did end up paying a mechanic. By learning how a car works and something about how to make repairs, I was better able to talk with my mechanic. I could understand what was wrong with my car, and I was able to make repair decisions more intelligently. As a bonus, with my grasp of details I could make sure that my mechanic was competent and honest.

This is the same state of affairs we seek when learning about our medical problems. Acquiring such knowledge through reading and discussions will not make us doctors, but it will allow us a deeper understanding that will lead to better decisions. It will let us see more clearly the thought process behind our medical care, and reinforce confidence in our caregivers.

So remember that you are not a doctor. Do not expect to treat yourself or know the pros and cons of each option. But also remember that your own medical knowledge is one of your most valuable tools for good medical decisions, a tool worth cultivating and developing.

(*Author's Note:* Even if you *are* a physician, you cannot be your own doctor. First, it is unlikely that your expertise lies in your own disease. Second, even if you are your own expert, you don't have the objective distance required for a healthy assessment of potentially painful choices.

Use your special knowledge, but don't try to escape the normal need to lean on your doctors for help.)

Don't doctor yourself.

USE YOUR DOCTOR AS A DOCTOR

Yes, doctors are nowadays more like advisors than benevolent parents. Yes, the authority of the doctor is being challenged by our desire for involvement in our medical decisions. And yes, economic pressure and social change have turned medicine into more of a business than ever before.

But there is still something special, something out of the ordinary, about the doctor.

That "something" is the relationship between doctor and patient, a relationship like no other. It is formed from the promise made to care for another, and the trust in that promise. It is a sacred relationship thousands of years old that survives today despite the twisted assaults from managed care and malpractice attorneys.

The impact of the doctor-patient relationship is felt as much by the doctor as the patient. For being a doctor is an intimate activity, formed from face-to-face conversations and a delivery of touch between two people. No human being can play this doctor's role and feel immune to the weighty obligation to that other person. No one, no matter what the economic pressures, can look another in the eye and ignore the ethical responsibility for the welfare of that other. It is as tangible as breathing, money be damned.

There are some doctors who perform their tasks mechanically. But even the coldest of doctors are human, and even the most sterile of exam rooms cannot prevent the foothold of the intimate bond between doctor and patient. Doctors feel and live their old, sacred vows, even if they are at times just a glimmer behind the business of medicine.

So as you use your doctor as a source of medical information and perspective, be aware that he or she is also a source of human concern and compassion. The advice you receive, unlike the dispassionate suggestions of a textbook, comes from the heart. Yes, the doctor is an advisor; but a special, irreplaceable advisor with your interests in mind.

Your doctor is still your doctor.

THE USE OF DOCTORS—RECAP

There will be plenty of times when your doctor will tell you what to do, and you will do it. This is normal and good. But we have crossed a line in our thinking about doctors, and there is no turning back. The doctor is no longer the final authority. He or she is now just another resource.

But what a resource, and how worthy of special treatment! The doctor is your best provider of medical fact, perspective, and advice. He or she is your advocate, ethically bound to look out for your best interests no matter what. You are still in control of your own medical future, and the quality of your decisions still depends on the quality of your medical knowledge. But the doctor's perspective and advice remain your most powerful tool for making your medical decisions.

Use it well.

Cherish the doctor.

—HOW TO INTERPRET YOUR DOCTOR—

The conversation you have with your doctor is not an ordinary conversation. True, information is being transmitted about a particular subject (you). And true, there is the usual assortment of nuances, half comments, and body language that embellish any discussion. But an interpretation of these nuances that is too relaxed or too casual can have a significant impact on your health. In this section, I'll give a few examples where close attention to how the doctor communicates will pay off.

BEWARE POLLYANNA

Joe K. is a 45-year-old car salesman who is considering eye surgery to improve his vision. After a few weeks of hesitation, he finally made an appointment at an eye clinic he had learned about from a radio advertisement. The doctor examined Joe's eyes, explained the surgical procedure, and concluded with, "You'll be just fine. We do a lot of these and your vision will be perfect!"

Marla and Bill M. were married two years ago, and are now ready for a family. At a recent visit to their doctor, they were overjoyed to learn that Marla was indeed pregnant and that their wish for a child would come true. Their enthusiasm was so contagious that the doctor himself was beaming as he scheduled an ultrasound and assured them that her pregnancy would of course be completely normal. Later that evening, Marla wondered to Bill, "Why do we need the ultrasound if the doctor said everything would be okay?"

Both Joe and Marla had cause to reflect on their doctor's comments. Since Joe is a cagey car salesman, he is naturally alert and suspects any hint of deception. A red light went off in his head when he heard the doctor's promise of perfect vision, since in his heart he knew that no one can guarantee a good outcome. Marla, on the other hand, is more trusting and less worldly than Joe. But she is not naive, and realized that the doctor would not have ordered the ultrasound test if there was truly no chance of a problem with her pregnancy. Both Joe and Marla knew better than to trust these Pollyanna promises.

It is difficult for any person to be the bearer of bad news. We enjoy bringing the happiness of good news far more than unearthing sadness with gloomy predictions. Doctors are no exception. We would much rather give you a clean bill of health than tell you that we have discovered an incurable cancer in your body. Even so, we are trained to be more objective, to deliver the bad news with the good, without flinching.

But doctors are people too, and occasionally a lapse of attention will allow unrealistic promises to break through. Rarely, the reasons may be sinister, as when the doctor is more interested in the surgery than the patient. Or the reasons may be due to indifference, as when the risks seem old hat to the doctor who has seen them a thousand times. More commonly, doctors simply want to give you good news rather than bad. Like Marla's obstetrician, they may find themselves caught up in the moment, making reassurances they cannot guarantee.

Small Pollyannaisms are common within medicine. How often have we heard, "This will only hurt a little bit"? Fortunately, the times you hear more serious Pollyannaisms from doctors are rare. But when you do, beware. Beware of absolute promises of good outcomes and of happy endings. Beware of "everything will be okay." Beware of undiluted optimism, because, as you've learned, good decisions require hearing both the good and the bad. A promise of a great outcome may make you feel good, but it can lead you astray from critical thinking. And it can sabotage the decision process that you have worked so hard to cultivate.

So when you hear these promises, push harder. Push to hear the bad predictions, the potential problems and complications. You may not want to; it is more comfortable to hear good news than bad. But you need to hear a balanced truth, not a pleasant fairy tale.

Beware "everything will be fine."

FACTS, OPINIONS, AND VALUE JUDGMENTS

Just as doctors are important sources of information, they are also key sources of the opinions we need to interpret the thousands of facts behind our medical decisions. For example, after your doctor informs you about the different drugs for the treatment of your asthma, you expect to hear his or her opinion as to which combination of drugs would be best for you. It is only natural to expect your doctor to be a source of medical advice as well as medical fact.

But it is equally natural to take the next step, to look to doctors for advice on how these medical interventions should fit into our lives. For example, a doctor may choose a medication for an elderly patient based partly on its ease of use in an attempt to avoid a confusing medicine schedule. Or your doctor may suggest that you send your recuperating mother to a rehabilitation hospital rather than taking care of her at home, since home care can be difficult. These are issues in which your doctor's wisdom can shine.

But these types of decisions are based on value judgments, not hard facts. Some elderly patients may prefer more complex medications for other reasons, and some families are well able to take care of their own at home. These are subjective choices, with no right or wrong answers. Although your doctor can provide a valuable perspective, in the end it is only your opinion that matters. These are decisions more of lifestyle and preference than of fact.

So as you discuss your decisions with your doctors, try to be aware of which issues are those of fact and which are value judgments. Listen to your doctor's perspective, for it is borne of years of experience. But realize that no one knows the complexity of your life as you do, and no one else can attach the proper value to each of your choices. It is up to you to make your own value judgments.

Don't confuse facts with advice.

EXPECT A SPECTRUM

Just as there are many types of people, there are many types of doctors. Some are expert in the technical aspects of medicine but are rather short on personality. Others have more basic skills but possess a bedside manner inspiring euphoric confidence. Some are timid, some are overconfident. Some like to talk, some like to listen. There are all types.

I might be criticized for this admission, since doctors are supposed to be all things to all people. We are all supposed to have the technical genius of Einstein and the tender compassion of a saint. But this of course cannot be true of any person. Don't expect it from your doctor.

It is wise to accept these differences and expect to benefit in different ways from different doctors. When talking with a brilliant surgeon, you might value the safety of his expert surgical skill without expecting the spiritual comfort that seems to pour from your family doctor. A discussion with your enthusiastic ophthalmologist who loves to talk about ways to improve your vision might be balanced by advice from another eye doctor who carefully listens to you to determine if contact lenses will fit into your lifestyle.

So don't expect each doctor to be all things. Don't judge your doctor harshly for not being both a saint and a genius. Instead, use each of your doctors for their strengths, allowing each to complement the other to match your medical needs. Take the best of what each of your doctors has to offer, and blend all these voices into your best medical decision.

Each doctor is different.

DOCTORS WITH HAMMERS

What will you hear if you ask a surgeon for advice on how to treat a disease? Other things being equal, you'll probably be told to have surgery.

And what will you hear if you ask an internist for advice? Probably treatment based on medications. To a man with a hammer, the world is a nail.

To be fair, patients are not referred to specialists unless there is reason to think there is need of the specialist's skill. No one makes it to the endocrinologist unless a referring doctor believes there is a problem with hormones, and the endocrinologist therefore expects to treat such diseases. Nails are generally sent to hammers.

But there is a danger to this type of thinking. Once someone believes that you have a surgical problem, it is very difficult for others to think anything else. Social psychologists call this the *anchor effect*; once a solution to a problem is proposed, subsequent solutions tend to be similar. It is difficult to break the mold.

So as you talk with your doctors, realize that each will propose solutions with which they are familiar. Remember to consider all your options, talk with different doctors, and keep an open mind.

Don't seek a hammer unless you're a nail.

MULTIPLE DOCTORS AND CAPTAINS

If you've read this far, you've learned that it is wise to consult with more than one doctor. The danger of this strategy is that you can get lost between the cracks, receiving different types of advice with no overall coordination. For that reason, I want to reiterate what we said in chapter three: You must have a captain. It is essential that you choose one doctor to coordinate your care, to provide a big picture, and to help you sort through all the advice. To do otherwise is to become lost in an uncharted medical ocean.

Find a captain for your medical ship.

—THE MYTH OF INFORMED CONSENT—

Ben and JoAnn H. are pleasant, middle-aged people who were sent to a surgeon after discovering that Ben's abdominal pain was caused by gallbladder disease. They are now sitting together in the surgeon's office, listening as he explains a few details of the surgery and gives them a date for the operation. After shaking their hands and bidding farewell, the surgeon leaves the room and a nurse enters to have Ben sign the required forms. She shows Ben the informed consent, a document containing a list of possible complications that can be caused by the operation. She explains these risks to Ben and his wife and has Ben sign at the bottom. Now that they know something about the pros and cons of the operation, Ben and JoAnn feel glad they have been well informed.

But they shouldn't.

The informed consent that we all must sign before any operation or other procedure is a document designed to protect us from certain abuses of power regarding information exchanged in the past between doctors and patients. In those times, more than a few patients received operations they did not agree to or for which they were inadequately educated. And it was considered the standard of care to deliberately withhold medical information from the patient, as it was simply none of his or her business.

But modern times have rightfully changed that state of affairs, and every doctor is now both ethically and legally bound to document the potential risks of a procedure to the patient before the operation. Standard lists of risks have been formulated, and the signing of these informed consents is a required preoperative ritual.

The problem is that informed consent is all too often a legal obligation and has no real meaning. The forms themselves are printed en masse, clearly not tailored for each specific patient. And the list of possible complications is so lengthy that it seems to be constructed more to avoid lawsuits than to provide intelligent information. When these impersonal forms are given to us by a nurse for our signatures in the doctor's absence, it is no wonder that we view informed consent as just another meaningless requirement.

And so I find myself commonly in the following predicament. I will explain each and every risk of an operation to my patients, as required by the informed consent doctrine. At the end of this long litany, the patient and his or her family will look at me and say, "Okay, that's great. Now tell us what you really think." They have realized that informed consent has deteriorated into a legal obligation, instinctively knowing that we have been transformed into legal adversaries, at least for a few moments. They are really saying to me, "Come on now, we know you just have to say all that so you won't be sued. Be a real doctor and tell us what you *really* think of the operation, and what we should look out for." And so I do.

My point is that your decision process should not be based on the legality of informed consent. It is true that you should understand that each of the listed complications can occur, and that you should ask about any that concern you or catch your eye. But the real data you need to make your decisions must come from honest, meaningful, and individual conversations between yourself and your doctor. Anything less is just another blank form.

Informed consent is not information.

THIRTEEN

When Doctors Disagree

"Who shall decide, when doctors disagree...?"

"Like doctors thus, when much dispute has past,
We find our tenets just the same at last."
—Alexander Pope, *Epistle III*

POPE WAS WRONG.

Still, his question was insightful. Who indeed should decide when doctors do not agree? Other doctors? Our friends? Ourselves?

But his answer was wrong, at least for modern times. When all the opinions are heard and when the smoke clears, our medical choices are not at all "just the same at last." Our choices are anything but the same: some lead to life and health, others do not.

And that is why the problem of doctors in disagreement is so terrifying. After weaving your way through a confusing maze of medical issues with the guidance of your trusted doctors, nothing could be more demoralizing than to find another doctor who disagrees with your plan. Does this mean your first doctor is an incompetent guide? Has he or she made some dreadful mistake? Or is it the second doctor who is mistaken? How do you tell?

The one who must decide is of course yourself. You must weigh the evidence, seek other advice as appropriate, and make the final decision when the experts cannot agree. This is a difficult task, fraught with uncertainty. Here are a few tips that will help.

You must decide when doctors disagree.

KNOW THE ISSUES

Suppose you discovered you had a disorder of calcium metabolism, a disorder you know little about. Suppose that one of your doctors advises taking medication right away to prevent further illness, but that another doctor thinks you should wait several years. What would you do?

My advice would be this: First learn all you can about your options and the reasons behind each doctor's thinking. Find out exactly what each doctor is advising, and why. Find out the pros and cons of their advice, and find out why they think what they do. Learn the issues before attempting to decide.

In other words, use the techniques you have learned in this book. Identify your options, identify the tradeoffs, discover the data in support of each view, and interpret the relevant numbers. It doesn't matter how many doctors are involved; the basic principles of medical decision making are the same. And don't be intimidated by having to talk with each of several doctors for this information; you already know how to do this! Although it may be awkward to use the doctor to hear a viewpoint rather than simply to follow his or her advice, this is the approach we have suggested even when your doctors agree. For your decisions are always your own, whether your doctors agree or not.

Decisions are decisions, no matter how many doctors.

KNOW YOUR DOCTORS

We said before that not all doctors are equal, and that you can obtain different benefits from different doctors. But now that your doctors disagree, you will have to assess these differences more critically. Because now you must choose which doctor to follow, or at least which advice to weigh more heavily in your thinking. You must choose a victor.

How you evaluate your doctors will depend on the type of problem you face. If you are trying to choose between two types of complex chemotherapies, the doctor with the greatest technical expertise might have more sway. A noted expert from a large cancer center will have more experience with these types of choices than your family doctor, even if your family doctor is a close friend and the expert is rather cold. On the other hand, if you are contemplating a surgery that might have a huge impact on your lifestyle and your family, a trusted family doctor who knows you well may offer more wisdom than the eloquence of experts. The right doctor is the one who fits the question.

So investigate your doctors. Investigate their credentials, make sure that they have expertise in your problem. Ask around to find out about their reputation, especially among friends who are health care workers. Don't be afraid to pose these questions to the doctors themselves and don't hesitate to travel to big medical centers for other opinions. Follow the most knowledgeable experts for technical advice, but remember that great wisdom can be found from doctors who know you well.

Check out your doctors.

SEEK OTHER OPINIONS

It is all well and good to evaluate credentials, but much of the time you will find your doctors to be equally matched. What do you do then?

One approach is to obtain a third or even fourth opinion. You might consult with other doctors in your city, or travel to several larger medical centers for further advice. The idea is not to use a third doctor as a "tie breaker," but rather, to gain a consensus opinion of what you should do. To that end, ask your doctors to talk with one another. You might be more convinced to take a particular medicine or have a particular surgery if four of your five doctors agreed that you should.

You may be reluctant to spend the time, energy, and money required to obtain multiple medical opinions. You will have to weigh the importance of your medical problems to decide whether these opinions are worth the effort. I would only suggest that you keep the long-term results in mind; it is often worth a dollar today for the peace of mind and good health of tomorrow.

Find more voices.

Lump Them Together

When doctors disagree, instead of thinking of the different opinions coming from many different experts, lump them all together. Pretend that all of these viewpoints have been explained to you by just one doctor. Forget that you are using a rather intimidating group of physicians and imagine you are consulting with a single, perhaps kindly, family doctor. He or she has given you some conflicting choices; how are you to decide?

The answer, of course, is to use the ideas and techniques presented earlier in this book. Follow the six steps of medical decision making you have learned. Make sure you understand your options and tradeoffs, and make sure you discover the appropriate data. You will need to gather up your beliefs, just as always, and to reflect on the personal meaning of your choices.

In other words, making decisions when the doctors cannot agree is really no different than making your decisions under the guidance of a single doctor. It may seem more frightening when even the experts cannot tell you what to do, but this is really the natural state of affairs. As always, your medical decisions must be made by you and must be based on your needs. It is your vote that is the most important tiebreaker when doctors don't agree.

Consolidate.

Rejecting the Doctor's Advice

If your doctors disagree with one another, you must choose which advice to follow. But then you will have to choose one doctor's advice, which means you will be rejecting the guidance of another. Some people are reluctant to do this, feeling that their doctor will become angry or offended. These patients may avoid their doctor rather than reveal their disputed decision, or worse, they may make their decisions to please the doctor. But remember that your doctor is there to guide you to a good decision, not to be your friend and not to be pleased by your decisions. Most doctors will respect your decisions and work to further your medical care, even if they do not fully agree with your plan. And at times you may choose a particular doctor to serve as your "captain," even if he or she does not fully agree with your choices.

So don't worry about what your doctors will think of you if you act against their advice. Good doctors will respect your responsible decision, even if they do not agree.

Be true to yourself, not your doctor.

Part IV
Deciding for Others

FOURTEEN

Deciding for Friends and Family

ALTHOUGH WE MAKE most of our medical decisions for ourselves, we are occasionally in the position of having to decide for others. We may be required to make decisions for our children, for parents who can no longer manage their own affairs, or for a recently disabled spouse. But responsibility for others is a frightening burden, so that making decisions for others is even more stressful and disturbing than making them for ourselves

Most of the time we are asked to simply help someone make a medical decision rather than make their medical decision ourselves. Husbands and wives consult each other about medical matters, children consult their parents, and friends consult friends. It is human nature to seek the counsel of others for important decisions. All of us, sooner or later, will play the role of the decider's helper.

In extreme cases, we may be called upon to do more than merely provide advice: we may be asked to actually make an important medical decision for a friend or family member. Adult children of elderly parents are often in this situation, as are friends of those too ill to decide for themselves. The responsibility given to us in these settings can be frightening and confusing.

What, then, is appropriate? Should we be aggressively directive, instructing the other person in explicit detail? Or should we be passive, offering advice only when asked and never pushing for any particular solution? Should we freely express our opinions, or should we hold our tongue? And how do we know what to decide if the other cannot speak?

The answers to these questions depend on the nature of the relationship between you and the other person. It may be appropriate for a husband to direct the medical care of his wife of forty years, especially if he has been the major decision maker in their relationship. It is less appropriate for a casual friend to urge your doctors to withhold painful but lifesaving medical treatment. Although universal rules for advising others do not exist, the type of relationship between the two people seems to be the most critical factor.

(I will assume that there are no legal issues preventing you from making these decisions, as it is not my intent to address legal matters. Likewise, I will assume that your assistance to this other person is ethically appropriate. Though important, these legal and ethical matters are beyond the scope of this book.)

Deciding for another depends on your relationship with the other.

THE THOUGHTS OF OTHERS

The *second* greatest handicap you face when helping others with their medical decisions is that you cannot read their minds. You cannot know their preferences unless they can tell you, and you cannot unerringly guess which choices would make them happy. You must rely on your relationship with that person to intuitively give the right advice, as a pilot navigates through a storm using instruments.

You may be wondering: If my inability to read minds is my second greatest handicap I face when deciding for others, what is my *first, and greatest,* handicap? In my opinion, it is the fact that even though you cannot read minds, you probably think you can.

We saw this problem when we discussed friends and family as sources of medical advice. People tend to believe that others agree with their own likes, dislikes, and opinions. The teenager who plays loud music believes that others will not mind listening, and those who drink feel that most others also enjoy alcohol. Social psychologist Gilovich discusses more examples in his book *How We Know What Isn't So*, and tells us the name for this phenomenon: the *false consensus effect*.

Just as your friends might believe they know your thoughts, you too may labor under the handicap that you know the preferences and beliefs of those you are helping. In some cases, you may be correct. Husbands and wives often know each other so well that one can make decisions for the other with complete comfort. But most other relationships are not endowed with this degree of intimacy. Although you might believe that your ill friend shares your fear of surgery or your wish to live no matter what, you may be wrong. You cannot read minds.

So as you help your friends and family to make their medical decisions, remember that they do not share your every opinion. Listen carefully to their beliefs and try to work within *their* viewpoint of the world. When they are unable to tell you their thoughts, use what you know about them to imagine what they might want for themselves. You may not always be absolutely correct, but you will be acting as a true friend.

You are not a mind reader.

RELATIONSHIP DYNAMICS

Katherine S. is a 54-year-old woman with an adult son Rick who requires continuing renal dialysis because of damage to his kidneys suffered long ago. Rick must spend several hours twice a week connected to the dialysis machine at the hospital, and has suffered a variety of surgical procedures and infections related to his illness over the years. Rick and his mother have always faced these medical challenges together, so that although Rick lives independently, they are as close as a mother and son can be.

After seeing the doctor for some fluttering feelings in his chest, Rick has learned that he is in danger of sudden death because of a problem with the firing pattern of his heart. There are two treatments. The first is a direct surgical modification of his heart, likely to be successful but risky. The second is treatment with medications, only a little less successful but likely to complicate his dialysis. The right decision is not clear.

Rick and his mother discuss his options in detail, as they have always done. He uses her as a sounding board, and she helps him find the medical information they need from books and from the Internet. They search for a comfortable decision as a team.

One night while at a friend's house for dinner, Rick and Katherine are again discussing his medical problems and options. Their friend listens quietly for a while, then looks Rick intensely in the eye and says, "You really should decide this for yourself. You're an adult now."

On the way home, Rick and his mother are quiet as they consider their friend's comment. True, Rick is a self-sufficient adult. But he and his mother have always solved his medical problems together with no smothering feelings of dependence. Should they stop now? Should Rick make his decisions alone? They are thoughtful and a bit confused.

I disagree completely with their friend. True, adults should be responsible for making their own decisions, but everyone obtains advice from others in their own particular way. It makes no sense for Rick to change how he consults with his mother just because he faces a new medical problem. Their relationship has served them well for many years, and to choose a new pattern would be arbitrary, painful, and perhaps harmful.

This principle holds for most families and for most groups of friends. Our ways of relating with one another do not change suddenly because of a crisis. If one family member has been dominant for years, that same person will likely play a major role during a new medical crisis. Spouses who bicker over daily decisions will argue over their medical decisions. And friends who lean on each other for advice will need each other during illness.

The patterns of our lives have evolved for many years, serving us in ways that may be subtle and unclear. Those same patterns will continue to be of use to us while making medical decisions. Don't expect to change the way you think and relate to others when a new medical problem comes along; your old ways are familiar, easier, and probably much better than anything you could imagine.

Don't change who you are.

FIFTEEN

Deciding for Children

THE SADDEST MOMENT in my neurosurgical career occurred when I watched a 3-year-old boy die quietly early one morning in the arms of his mother in our intensive care unit. He had been declared brain-dead following a head injury the night before, an injury so grievous that surgery could not help. With the family's agreement, and with all ethical i's dotted and t's crossed, the senior neurosurgeon and I made ready to turn off the ventilator and end his life. But the boy's mother wanted to hold her son while his body died, and she did so with such moving dignity that my colleague and I could only stand by in respectful silence as the ventilator sighed to a halt.

Why was this event so especially sad? As a neurosurgeon, I had seen enough carnage and trauma and human tragedy to fill an encyclopedia. Perhaps it was because at that time I had small children of my own, or perhaps it was because we were so helpless to save that boy and spare that mother the agony of witnessing her child's death. But I think that the reason I will never forget those few moments is that illness is particularly and painfully tragic in children.

General Thoughts: Anxiety and Trust

There is something about struggling with a child's illness that touches us unlike illness in adults. Perhaps it is because children touch us with their vulnerability and special type of innocence. This is especially so with our own children, where the effects of disease magnify our already acute protective parental instincts. No medical situation provokes more anxiety and despair than those that hurt children.

This anxiety is normal and unavoidable. It will always be there no matter what kind of medical problem your child faces. It is a required part of your emotional landscape, something to be accepted rather than fought. This means that making decisions for your children will be a lot harder and more uncomfortable than making decisions for yourself.

You may therefore find yourself more demanding than usual, perhaps pushing your doctors into quick action while at the same time needing extra time to make firm decisions. You may wonder if you are being taken seriously by your doctors and nurses, and you may feel powerless to stop a train of events that only seems to threaten your child even more.

The best way to make it through this tough period is to make sure that you trust your doctor. It is essential that you feel that your doctor listens to you, responds to your concerns appropriately, and has the best interests of your child at heart. Only then can you rest easy with the knowledge that your doctor is acting as your partner to protect and nurture the health of your child. No one can tell you how to establish this trust, or how to tell if your doctor meets these important needs for you. But just as you find people to trust in other facets of your life, you can do the same with physicians.

A good physician will not always agree with you, even though he or she will always listen and try to understand. Suppose, for example, your child has leukemia and develops a runny nose. You demand that steroids be started at once, but your doctor, thinking that your child has a simple cold, wishes to persuade you otherwise. Here is where the trust you have developed is crucial, as it is in negotiating any decisions for your child with your doctor.

The methods we have discussed earlier in this book for making decisions for ourselves can also be used to reach medical decisions for our children. The same steps apply: Identify your options and trade-offs, discover numbers, gather your beliefs, and contemplate the meaning of the decision. In addition, it is crucial that you develop a trust in your doctor so that your thinking is not clouded by the intense anxiety that naturally accompanies all illness in children.

Find a doctor you can trust with your children.

WHEN PARENTS DISAGREE

Medical decisions for children are often complex and usually made during moments of anxiety and stress. It is therefore not surprising that parents are not always in full agreement. The decisions are difficult, the outcomes are unknown, and the possibility of even rare complications is frightening. Parents often argue about the smallest of decisions, since every detail seems so critical.

If the parents are separated or divorced, these disagreements can easily escalate to dangerous levels. Although the bond between separated parents can be strengthened by a medical crisis affecting their child, the conflicts of a divorce can easily leak out, magnifying the anger between parents to create arguments having more to do with old resentments than with new medical problems. Reaching a good medical decision in this atmosphere is almost impossible.

Most of the time, differences between parents can be resolved with discussion, compromise, and perhaps with the doctor's help. After all, no matter how bitter the previous arguments have been, both parents want what is best for the child. But occasionally, conflict cannot be resolved even after much conversation. For these cases, prompt professional counseling is probably the best alternative. The goal here is not to solve the problems of the parents, but to head everyone in the same direction so as not to injure the child.

The child is the one who is sick.

DOES THE CHILD GET A VOTE?

Trish M. is a charming 13-year-old girl who unfortunately was recently found to have a small brain tumor. She seems perfectly healthy and does well in school. Trish and her parents came to my office to discuss surgery to remove the tumor. Several times during the conversation, I was a bit disturbed to hear the family say, "Well, it's really her decision. Trish, what do you want to do?" And at this point, Trish would chew her gum, shrug her shoulders, look at the wall, and mumble, "I don't know."

Children are people, too, and deserve a degree of choice in their lives. But how much, and for what types of medical decisions? For Trish, my opinion was that the decision for or against brain surgery was simply too serious for her alone, and I made sure the family was more involved than they appeared to be at first. But it is difficult to give general rules that apply to all circumstances.

Parents of babies, infants, and small children will obviously be the ones making the medical decisions. Once a decision is made, however, I believe that even young children should be told about the decisions at a level appropriate to his or her understanding.

The issue is less clear for older children, for example, those between 10 and 15 years old. Some children may have strong opinions regarding their own treatment, and families vary tremendously in how much autonomy they allow their children. For most medical decisions, it is my opinion that the parents should have the major vote in this age group, even if long conversations are required. But not all families would agree.

Teenagers, as we all know, can be problematic. Some teenagers are quite mature, with decision-making powers equal to adults, and their opinions should probably be given strong weight. Other teenagers are immature and rebellious, so that family or physician input may be crucial. Again, your doctor may be able to guide you here and professional counseling may be helpful.

You must decide who will decide.

Part V
Special Problems

SIXTEEN

Pitfalls

SAMUEL JOHNSON defined a pitfall as "a pit dug and covered, into which a passenger falls unexpectedly." The oldest pitfalls may have been used to trap birds, but later uses included the capture of tigers, elephants, and even the occasional rhinoceros. Modern pitfalls await us as we struggle with our medical decisions, and, like Johnson's passengers, we may find ourselves trapped unexpectedly. This chapter will give you a map of the most common pitfalls so you can safely skirt them.

SOME DECISION DON'TS

One of the most helpful findings taught to us by those who study decision making is that a few common mistakes seem to be committed again and again while making important decisions. Some of these are summarized in the very useful book *Decision Traps* by J. Edward Russo and Paul Schoemaker, and some have been alluded to earlier in this book. Here are some particularly common mistakes to keep in mind when making medical decisions.

Don't jump right in. The heroes in our movies always seem to know what to do right away, but life is not a movie. Most of the time, even if we think we know our minds and know what we need to do, it is better to wait before the final commitment. Give yourself some time to gather data and to ruminate over all the angles, or, as we said earlier, sleep on it.

Don't be overconfident. This is related to the mistake above. Admit to yourself you don't know everything. Think carefully even if your thoughts seem sure. An ounce of prevention here is worth a pound of cure.

Don't agonize once you have made your decision. Trust yourself. If you have been careful and thoughtful, you will make the best possible decision that you can. No decision is free of risk (as we have said again and again!), and it is better to accept your final decision than to agonize too long over the details.

Don't stop at just one way of looking at the data. We discussed this earlier when we saw that a 10% mortality rate could also be considered to be a 90% survival rate. These differing viewpoints (called *frames* by the social psychologists) can dramatically alter our decision process. Don't let them. Turn the data upside down, backward, and sideways to see all the different angles. Don't get caught with just one way of looking at the decision. Think outside the frame.

Don't be fooled by flimflam. Be skeptical. Learn to distinguish advertisements from balanced reports. Don't be overly swayed by testimonials, no matter how much you want to believe in a good outcome. Don't take any authority as the last word. Be skeptical (have I said that before?).

Don't put too much trust in group decisions. Although it is human to take comfort in the advice of others, social psychologists know that groups of people often make poor decisions. Listen to your friends, listen to your family, but take the decisions that come from group discussion with a grain of salt.

Don't forget the past. Our happiness with our past decisions can be invaluable guidance to the decisions of the future. Don't make the same mistake twice.

Don't be ruled by convenience. Ours is a convenience society, ruled by fast action and inexpensive solutions. Unfortunately, your medical care may not be so easy. You may be faced with the choice of receiving your medical care inexpensively from the local clinic, or pursuing a more effective but costly consultation with far-away experts. These decisions are difficult because our resources are finite, but remember that it is the final result that is important. Don't be hemmed in by convenience and insurance. Do what you have to do.

REMEMBERING IT ALL

Stephan M. is a 38-year-old computer programmer who went to his doctor because of abdominal pain that awakened him at night for about two weeks. He felt fine otherwise, but his doctor ran some tests, one thing led to another, and a small, deeply placed tumor was found lying just next to his spine at the level of his belly button. On hearing this news, Stephan and his wife, who is also a programmer, were understandably frightened, and not at all comforted by their doctor's recommendation to see a cancer surgeon.

Nor did the cancer surgeon do much to slow the mounting terror in both Stephan and his wife. After asking some questions and looking at Stephan's studies, the surgeon confirmed the fact that indeed there was a tumor, and that it might be malignant. The only way to tell would be a biopsy, but in any case, the tumor would need to be removed.

You can imagine the panic in Stephan's mind when he heard these words. It was as if he were caught in a powerful vortex of bad news from which he could not escape. He continued to talk with the surgeon, but his mind was tuning out, and it became more difficult to focus and remember things. His responses and questions became automatic, as if they came from someone else.

The surgeon spent about an hour with Stephan and his wife, explaining what might happen. The explanation was filled with medical terms and seemed complicated. If the biopsy showed malignancy, then Stephan might need some chemotherapy before his surgery. If the tumor could be removed with free margins (i.e., if there was no tumor left at either end of the operative wound), then he would not need radiation therapy unless the degree of malignancy was high. The degree of malignancy (or grade) would be determined in the laboratory once the tumor was removed. If free margins could not be achieved, Stephan would probably need radiation, and maybe even chemotherapy. The danger of the tumor growing back depended on free margins, and the danger of the tumor spreading to other organs depended on the grade of malignancy.

The surgeon went on to say that his partner, Dr. X., actually had more experience with these types of tumors and that it would be in Stephan's best interest to continue with this second surgeon. Dr. X. would be in town for a week but was then leaving on vacation. The original surgeon then introduced Stephan and his wife to his nurse, who began scheduling all of the various appointments. She told Stephan that the nurse for Dr. X. would be taking over, but that she, too, was out of town for two weeks and that a third nurse would be covering for her until that time. Stephan and his wife, grateful for the help but terrified beyond comprehension, smiled and mumbled their thanks as they received the paperwork necessary for all of the arrangements.

That next day, Stephan and his wife were driving to work, a bit calmer as they discussed his medical plans.

"So, did he say I'll need surgery for sure?" Stephan asked.

"Which doctor, the first doctor? I thought he said you just needed a biopsy." His wife seemed annoyed.

"No," Stephan said, frowning and trying to remember, as he kept his eyes on the road. " I thought I was supposed to get chemotherapy first, then surgery. But I forget what he said about radiation."

His wife looked sharply at him and said, "I thought Dr. X. said that they were going to do a biopsy and then decide about chemotherapy. But what did he say about surgery?"

"Well, I guess we'll have to call them and see. Was it Dr. X. who is out of town?"

She thought hard for a second and replied, "I think so. Which of those nurses do you think we should call? I didn't catch which of them is handling our case."

What happened to them? Stephan and his wife are intelligent people, survivors in the competitive world of computer programming, and their doctor spent more than an hour with them explaining the medical issues. Yet neither Stephan nor his wife could recall what had been said, or what the medical issues were, or even whom to call for clarification. The reason, of course, is that it is nearly impossible for anyone to muster the mental focus required to assimilate new information during times of stress, especially when the medical information involves complex options and a multitude of doctors, nurses, and tests. In fact, it has been shown that people are rather poor at remembering details of even ordinary conversations. And since medical information is particularly stressful and commonly explained in several sessions spread out over time, it is no wonder that confusion is the rule rather than the exception. So no matter how smart you are, what happened to Stephan and his wife can easily happen to you.

I have a simple solution for this problem that is as effective as it is anticlimactic: Write it down. Accept the fact that your mental faculties will not be operating at full throttle during these difficult conversations, bring a pen, and write down who said what and when. In fact, I would recommend that you keep an information log, either in a special blank book from the stationery store or on paper kept in a special folder. Write the date of the visit or phone call, whom you are talking with, and what they say. Write everything down even if the details seem obvious; they won't seem so clear later. Write it down as they say it or immediately afterward, and don't be afraid to ask them to repeat or clarify the information; they won't mind at all, really. Keep your notes neat and take the time to make your handwriting legible, because you will be reading these notes perhaps months in the future when your memory of the conversation is dim. Keep this log in a handy place, and *bring it with you* every time you see every medical professional, not just the doctors.

You may not be able to keep such a log when you first hear disturbing news. Your mind may be elsewhere, distracted by the normal stress of those moments. But after the shock wears off, when you regain your bearings, start writing.

The rewards for this simple task are huge. You will have a record of medical recommendations and of the thought processes of your doctors that you can review at any time. You will also have a record of whom you are to see, whom you are to call, and when the various tests and procedures are to take place. Regardless of how you use your doctor's advice, your log will be of immense benefit to you as you struggle with your medical decisions.

In fact, you might consider keeping other logs for other related issues. Keeping a "to do" list and brief logs for insurance issues (who promised what and when), for medical articles, for hotel arrangements, for medical records, and for wills may be helpful. The complexity of your medical situation will determine how much of this you need, although the important thing is to keep the logs updated as you go along and bring them with you to all your medical events and appointments.

As I suggested earlier, I highly recommend that you keep a special personal log, consisting of your thoughts and emotions as you go through the process of coping with your medical problem. For some people, writing down these intimate thoughts helps focus their thinking, while for others the act of writing can serve as a catharsis. In any case, I believe that writing down your thoughts, even briefly or cryptically, will greatly assist you in each of our six steps of decision making, and especially in the contemplation of meaning.

One final tip: Keep your personal log handy, day and night. Or keep a piece of paper in your pocket to jot down your ideas when they come. Insights do not arrive conveniently on schedule, and you will want to capture them in their native form as they occur.

No one can remember the shortest conversation. Write it down.

INSURANCE AND FINANCIAL MATTERS

So far, I have encouraged you to make your medical decisions without regard to worries of money or insurance. But once you have emerged with a decision between your teeth, you are likely to find that some or all of your intended medical plans are not covered by your insurance. Or more disturbing, you may find that you cannot possibly afford your most thought-out and cherished decisions.

Let me make an observation: Patients who have money or good-quality insurance will get better medical care than those who do not.

Don't be offended. I am not saying that this state of affairs is right, or that we should not work to change it. I am only pointing out that this is the current state of reality. Some would deny the truth of this admission, although a short visit to any large hospital would persuade anyone to the contrary. Others recognize the profound effect of money on medical care, but believe that these inequities will soon be remedied by Medicare or the HMOs. You can deny it or be philosophical, but like it or not, those with money or insurance are medically privileged just as the wealthy enjoy nicer cars, homes, and vacations. It is a fact of life.

And the relationship between money and quality of life is a fact with which we are intimately familiar. We are accustomed to searching for the best bargain for a car, or for homeowner's insurance. We are accustomed to budgeting for groceries or college expenses. We are accustomed to the work required to maximize the benefits from our incomes. Medical expenses are no different, and they too must fit into our existing financial circumstances. It does no good to cry that medical care is essential or to take these limitations personally. Our society and the world we live in is structured by money.

So when financial limitations threaten to block your medical decisions, you will have to assess your resources and make some difficult choices. We will divide our discussion into circumstances which are impossible, difficult, and inconvenient.

When It's Impossible
It may be that it is simply financially impossible for you to obtain the care that you have chosen. You may be without insurance, or your insurance company may flatly refuse to pay. But it is still worthwhile to go through the six steps, to research your options and think about your choices. Because in most cases, you will have access to your second choices—perhaps surgery at a smaller hospital or the use of older medications. And remember, knowing about your disease and its treatment gives you a sense of control and security even if your actual options are limited. Rarely, it may be worth it to you to seek extreme measures, such as legal action or a local fund-raising effort for your medical care, but usually you will have to cut your losses and rethink your decisions.

When It's Difficult
If your first choice of care is possible but difficult, you also have some tough choices. Your choice of surgeon may require a payment of cash from you, or you may have to pay for long-term therapy without insurance benefits for many years. You will have to decide how much your

first choice is worth to you, and whether you want to assume an uncomfortable amount of debt or rely on relatives and friends. As you assess your options, don't forget that many public hospitals offer superb medical care, even if the accommodations are less than luxurious.

When It's Inconvenient

Finally, obtaining your medical choices may simply be inconvenient, because of added expense, travel, or time. In the long run, you will probably be happier accepting the inconvenience and attaining your first choice, but again, the decision is yours.

I do not have good answers for these problems. Inequities in medical services are painfully common, even if it is taboo to admit they exist or talk about the problem. But it is better to accept financial limitations as problems to be figured into your overall decision strategy than to court disaster by refusing to acknowledge that they exist at all until it is too late.

Like it or not, money is a problem.

WHAT IF YOU CAN'T DECIDE?

In an episode ("I, Mudd") of the classic TV series *Star Trek*, the character Spock confronts two evil androids who appear to be absolutely identical women. He deliberately chooses one of them as his favorite, explaining that he chose her because she was identical to her twin. The computer controlling the androids finds this logic to be so unfathomable that its circuits burn out, allowing Spock and his colleagues once again to save the universe.

Like Spock, we are sometimes confronted with two options that seem equally matched despite our best efforts at analysis and introspection. Two alternatives may have equal risks and rates of success, and may have equal but different meanings to us within our system of beliefs. Yet even after allowing time for our thoughts to mature, and after consulting friends and physicians, we may find that two very different alternatives are quite equally matched. How then can we decide?

If you find yourself in this quandary, I would suggest that you first review all your steps. Look again at the statistics, gather again your beliefs, and reexamine the meaning of the decision, since a true stalemate is quite rare. There is usually a glimmer of a hint that can point you in the direction of a decision.

But occasionally the stalemate is real, unyielding to your best contemplative efforts. In these cases, you must simply choose, even if it seems you are choosing at random. It may be that your unconscious mind will guide you, as hands are guided over a Ouija board to give prophecy, or as some patients who suffer blindness due to brain damage can nevertheless point to the correct answer during visual testing. Or it may be that once you make a choice, its consequences really sink in and confirm (or refute) your decision.

In either case, just relax, close your eyes, and choose. Like Spock, in a true stalemate you cannot completely lose.

Sometimes you've just got to choose.

SEVENTEEN

Special Decisions

OUR SIX-STEP PLAN gives you a comprehensive array of powerful tools for approaching virtually any type of medical decision. But some decisions deserve special consideration. Here we will take a close look at these unique situations and show you how you can handle them.

CHOOSING TO DO NOTHING

Your doctor has told you that you need surgery, and has explained three different operations that might be helpful. One has a risk of chronic pain, another has a high risk of death, and a third is extremely expensive. You don't like any of these alternatives, and wonder if you can choose to do nothing. Why not?

You always have the option of "doing nothing." After all, your doctors have no wish or power to run your life or to make you accept medical treatment. And "doing nothing" is frequently an attractive option, since it spares you from the risks of "doing something."

But you need to realize something important: "Doing nothing" is in fact doing something. By choosing to forgo all medical treatment, you are accepting the risks of the natural history of your disease. If you refuse treatment for your diabetes, you are at risk for the ravages of that disease upon your eyes or kidneys. If you decide to postpone surgery for a broken leg, you risk future malformation and pain. There is really no such thing as "doing nothing."

My point is that you should consider "doing nothing" as just another medical choice requiring your thoughtful consideration. You will have to discover the consequences of leaving your disease untreated just as you must learn the consequences of any other medical treatment. You will have to incorporate the choice to "do nothing" into your assessment of your beliefs and meanings as you use the six-step plan. "Doing nothing" is always a choice worth thinking about, as long as you realize that you are really doing something.

"Doing nothing" is doing something.

WHEN THERE ISN'T TIME

The most horrible medical decision that could ever confront anyone is that faced by victims of massive burns. These unfortunate people seem unharmed at first, but almost all die in the next few days from massive swelling and organ failure. In the first few hours, however, they have a choice: elect to have a breathing tube placed in their throat, in a heroic but probably futile effort to prolong life, or refuse the breathing tube to allow a few last words with their family before their airway inexorably closes. Facing such a choice seems starkly incomprehensible.

I hope your choices are never this grim. But you may face medical situations in which time is limited. Car accidents or gunshot wounds, for example, often require immediate surgery with no time for lengthy deliberation. And certain forms of cancer or heart disease can require definitive treatment within days. In these cases, all you can do is trust the doctors around you to do the right thing. In a way, these decisions are easy since you really have no choice.

At other times, you will have a real but limited opportunity to consider your choices. You may need to decide about treatment for a cancer growing so rapidly that time is of the essence, or you may want to decide about a surgery before your insurance ends. You may have time to use all of the techniques in this book, but not time enough to use them well.

When time is severely limited, your decisions will be intuitive guesses rather than deliberate plans. For it takes time to learn about your medical problems, time to gather your beliefs, and time to contemplate the meaning of your choices. You cannot hurry these processes, but only accept the answers that arise from a hasty formulation.

Because of those limitations, I have listed below an abbreviated version of our six steps tailored to those situations in which your time for decisions is brief. They constitute a "short form" for medical decision making and will be helpful when you must come to a decision within minutes or hours.

1. **Decide where to receive your care.** You may find yourself in a strange emergency room after a car accident, or you may be told by your own doctors that you need chemotherapy right away. In either case, you may want to be taken elsewhere, either to a larger medical center or to a hospital closer to home. It is imperative that you ask the risks of such a move and that you know the risks of delay. Your gunshot wound may be best treated by a large trauma center across town, but you may not survive the move itself. Or the three-week delay required for treatment at a far-away cancer center might prove to be lethal. Your doctors will advise you frankly, if not bluntly, in such circumstances.

    Once you decide whether to stay put or move, be content with your decision. You've made it under stress, with limited time and information, and it represents your best effort in trying times.

2. **Find your options.** This step is the same as always, except now there is limited time. Your best sources of information will be your doctors. Be prepared to find that your options might be limited to two or three choices.

3. **Find the tradeoffs.** Again, you will not have time to research the pros and cons of your choices. But ask your doctors specifically for this information.

4. **Read if you can.** You will obviously not be able to read if you are in an emergency room, but you may want to research some issues if

you have a few days to make your decisions. Stick to standard text-books and familiar Web sites; you don't have time to be fancy.

5. **Lean on your family.** Limited time means stressful time. You will be distracted by worries, and your thinking will not be calm or rational. Lean on your family, and listen to them carefully, for they can help you in these times when you need it most.

6. **Contemplate the meaning.** Don't leave out this step. Even a few minutes spent in contemplation of the potential consequences of your decisions can be valuable.

You can accomplish much even in a short amount of time. And, as before, it is important that you be satisfied with your decisions. It is the best you can do under extreme conditions.

The only real hedge against these urgent settings is to prepare for them in advance. You cannot anticipate every medical problem, but you can think about your beliefs and consider the meanings of various choices before medical problems arise. How do you feel about surgery? How much disability would you accept to prolong life? Would you rather be treated with medications or radiation? Such thoughts won't fully answer your concerns when problems arise, but it is always better to be prepared.

Do the best you can do when time is short.

DECIDING ABOUT MEDICAL TESTING

Most medical tests have little risk. A routine blood test or X-ray may be expensive or uncomfortable, but will not be life threatening. A few tests, however, such as an angiogram (a test in which dye is injected into an artery through a catheter) or a biopsy, do in fact carry a small risk and can be likened to a small operation. These deserve your attention as much as any important medical decisions.

You can approach these decisions just like any other, using our six steps. Some special questions to ask are these:

+ How will this test help discover my diagnosis?
+ What is the chance of success?
+ What is the risk of the test?

✦ And, most important: Will the test change how my disease is treated?

For example, you may be advised to undergo a cardiac angiogram to assess the health of your coronary arteries. This test will be used to determine whether you need a cardiac bypass, and if so, which vessels need attention. Such a test is obviously essential to your health, as long as the risk of the angiogram is lower than the risk of a future heart attack. On the other hand, a biopsy of a kidney tumor may be less essential if surgery for the tumor is planned regardless of the biopsy results. The risk of the biopsy may not be worth the benefits of early information.

You may be tempted on occasion to refuse routine blood tests or X-rays. Sometimes such a refusal makes sense; perhaps duplicate tests have been ordered, or you have improved and the tests are no longer necessary. A short discussion with your doctor usually resolves the issue. But as we discussed earlier, routine tests can become symbols of our fears and frustrations at being ill. Refusing the tests may then feel good but may also hinder your doctor's efforts. A discussion with your friends, family, and doctors often clears this up.

You can treat medical tests like any other medical intervention. You can read about them in books, find discussions on the Internet, and talk with your doctors. They deserve the careful attention that you give to all of your medical decisions.

There is one special problem with some tests; you may not want to know the results. For example, it is now possible to predict whether family members of patients with Huntington's disease will themselves develop the disease later in life. Because there is no treatment for this disease, and because its course is one of unremitting dementia, some would rather not know their fate. These are personal choices with few general guidelines.

Treat medical tests like any other treatment.

DECIDING TO PARTICIPATE IN EXPERIMENTAL TRIALS

Medicine is a conservative art. Despite labels of "cutting edge" and "advanced technique," most medical care is made from tried-and-true interventions that have withstood the test of time. Doctors want to stick with these treatments because they are dependable, and they are reluctant to try untested methods because of unknown dangers.

But newer and more effective treatments are always being invented, developed by innovative doctors and sought after by patients who want more than standard medicine. The most accepted way for these new methods to be tried is with an experimental trial. And that leads to our next decision: Should you or should you not participate in an experimental trial?

There are two ways to become part of an experimental trial. The first is to be offered this role by your doctors. They may explain that a new medication is being tested with certain theoretical advantages, or that a new surgery is being tried for your condition. The second way is for you to seek trials that you feel might be beneficial. Asking your doctors is of course one way to find new trials, and Web sites such as www.clinical trials.gov are sources of up-to-date lists. Patients who actively look for trials are often dissatisfied with their current medical care, such as the patient with cancer for whom treatment is not working.

There are certainly advantages of participating in a clinical trial. First, you may have access to a new and better treatment of your medical condition that is not otherwise available. You may receive better care and more attention than usual, since patients in trials are often hand picked and carefully followed. Some of your treatment may be free, especially if the trial is well funded. Finally, your participation may help doctors develop better medical methods that will benefit other patients like yourself in the future.

But there are distinct disadvantages of participation in clinical trials. You may find yourself assigned to the control group, in which you do *not* receive the new therapy being tested. In this case, your results will be used for comparison with other patients who do receive the new therapy. Even if you are treated with the new therapy, you might be chosen to receive a low dose rather than a high dose. And there may be unanticipated risks. After all, if everything were known about the new method, it would not require testing. You may be asked to travel or to return for more doctor visits than customary. Your insurance may refuse to pay for your treatment, since many companies will not pay for experimental trials. Finally, you may lose the participation of your own physician as the doctors in charge of the trial take over your care.

Be careful as you decide to participate. It is tempting to get swept away in the fanfare of scientific achievement, and equally tempting to ignore the possibility that you can be injured by your choices (we discussed our preference for believing in good results earlier). Make sure you understand all the details of the study and what will be required of you.

Participation in a clinical trial can have lifesaving benefits, making new therapies available to you that are otherwise unattainable. But make sure that these new therapies are right for you, and make sure you know all the rules.

Know the rules of the trial.

DECIDING ABOUT ALTERNATIVE TREATMENTS

I have to confess to a rather dim view of the "alternative treatments" that are now so popular. One reason for my view is exemplified by a recent patient at our hospital, who stopped her medicine to treat her brain tumor with a macrobiotic diet. Her tumor size doubled within a month, and shortly after that I read her obituary in the local newspaper.

But don't let my viewpoint anger you or put you off. I am willing to admit there may be benefits to some of the alternative treatments and to admit that many have not been thoroughly investigated. And I know that many standard medical treatments were once "alternative," and that many currently accepted conventional treatments will be discredited in the future.

Still, there can be some dangers to these alternative treatments.

First, there is little standardization and no regulation within this field. This means that quacks line up side by side with more reputable therapists, and you can't tell one from the other. Web sites such as www.quackwatch.com may help by exposing the worst of the charlatans, but you still need to beware.

Alternative treatments are also dangerous because they are so pleasant. Who would not rather be wrapped in warm herbal salts than undergo chemotherapy? The problem is that the risks and efficacy of medical therapies have little to do with the enjoyment of their experience. You wouldn't judge a book by its cover, so it makes no sense to make medical decisions based on the charm of the practitioner or the taste of the medicine.

Finally, alternative therapies can be dangerous if you completely reject the advice of your doctors or stop your standard treatment. It is vitally important that you tell your doctor if you adopt an alternative treatment and discuss whether to continue your standard treatment. Keeping your doctor in the dark can be lethal.

So as you consider whether to use alternative therapies, be careful. Learn as much as you can about them, and avoid quackery. Ask to see data, and be as skeptical as you would about a new surgery or new medication. Keep your doctor informed, and make sure you understand the consequences of altering your standard therapy. Your life depends on it.

Be careful.

WHEN THERE'S NO HOPE

There may be times in your illness when it seems you have no choices, when the illness you are fighting seems sure to win, and when there is no hope. While that is eventually true for all of us, it may be worthwhile to seek other choices when it seems to be happening to you. Talk frankly with your doctors, consult with the big medical centers, talk to friends, and use the Internet. You may find other opinions or alternatives that are worth pursuing.

But there will be a time for all of us when there is no more time, and death is inevitable. Just know that there are still choices to be made and roads to be traveled. Medicine has made great progress in helping people to achieve a death with dignity and without pain. While this topic is beyond the scope of this book, your doctor can provide guidance and expertise in these difficult but inevitable times.

There are always choices to be made.

Part VI
You've Made Your Decision; Now What?

EIGHTEEN

How to Know When Your Medical Decision Is Good

THE REAL-LIFE PRACTICE of making decisions is anything but automatic. Assessments of tradeoffs can be ambiguous, our belief system hazy, and we are all too often ambivalent about the meaning of our medical decisions. How then, at the end of this process, do we determine if our decision is a good one or if we need to agonize further?

As usual, it is helpful to start with some examples. David M. is a 65-year-old executive who loves his job to the exclusion of most other activities in his life. He is overweight, smokes cigarettes, and is more than a casual social drinker. He does not exercise regularly, or in fact, at all. Surprisingly, he is medically sophisticated and understands the risk factors for heart disease that he has allowed to creep into his life. But even though he has thought about it more than a little, he has not read much of the medical literature that would warn him about these risk factors he faces. Yet he remains willing to accept these risks in return for what he considers to be a happy lifestyle. And so he announces to me, almost jovially, that he has decided not to exercise, stop smoking or drinking, or watch his diet. It appears he has made up his mind about how he wants to live his life.

John D. is a 45-year-old man with a brain tumor that has fortunately been found to be benign. The decision with which he struggles is whether to treat this tumor with radiation or wait until the tumor grows (his doctors tell him that it may, or may not, remain the same size forever). He has read through eight medical books on the topic, skimmed over a hundred medical articles, and waded through innumerable Web sites offering advice for the treatment of his type of tumor. He has had long conversations with friends and consulted with six physicians. He is arguably the most well informed person on the face of the planet about this one medical issue. But he cannot decide, and he always changes his mind as soon as he thinks he has made a decision. He is in decision limbo.

TWO CRITERIA

These examples suggest two criteria that might tell us when our decisions are good. The first criterion is that of due diligence: A certain amount of toil and investigation and thought must be given to the decision for it to be satisfactory. No one, for example, would choose to have open-heart surgery without at least a moment's thought and some deep conversations with the doctor. In David's case, the thought behind his decision may not be as thorough as we might wish, even though he claims to have carefully considered his risk factors and their consequences. We might doubt that he has really thought hard beyond his own wishful thinking, or taken the trouble to know the actual numerical risks, or contemplated deeply what might happen to him. And so we might conclude that his decision is a poor one. On the other hand, if he has indeed thought deeply about his circumstances, then I would defend his decision as a good one (but only for him).

The case of John is just the reverse. John has put more deep thought into his medical problem than any other human being alive, but has absolutely no clue what decision would make him happy. This suggests the second of our criteria for a good decision: The decision must sit well with us in an intuitive way. We must be satisfied with our decision, even if the outcome is unclear.

Admittedly, this criterion is imprecise. What does "sit well" mean? What is intuitive? I believe that all of us have an intuitive, gut feeling of contentment when our decisions are right for us, a feeling that defies measurement but is nevertheless real and important. The way to achieve this feeling cannot be prescribed, and often occurs suddenly, as when the veracity of a decision "strikes" us right. Conversely, a well-reasoned decision is wrong if your feelings about it are of dread and anxiety. The six steps of medical decision making that you've learned are designed to prepare your mind for decisions that will be satisfying to your all-important intuition.

I would propose two criteria, therefore, for determining whether your decision is a good one.

1. Make sure that your investigation and introspection have been adequately thorough and intense. In particular, be sure that you have considered the pros and cons and made a reasonable attempt to find and use all available information.
2. Make sure that the decision makes sense to you at a gut level. In language we have used before, be sure that you are satisfied with the decision in light of the meaning that the decision has for you.

Imprecise as these criteria are, they are reasonable guideposts that you can trust to confirm your decisions or lead you to reexamine decisions that may prove to be wrong. And they can help you avoid needless painful agonizing once your decisions have been made.

You'll know a good decision when you see it.

CHANGING YOUR MIND

There will be times when you want to change your mind about your medical decisions. You may have made a careful review of all the data, or you may sit up in bed one night with an epiphany. No matter; you've changed your mind and you want to change your medical decision.

Changing your mind about medical decisions can be awkward. Surgeries must be rescheduled, medicines must be changed, and discussions must be held with doctors. Many patients are reluctant to change their plans, fearing to inconvenience the entire medical system. They rethink their changes of heart, rationalizing their decision not to change out of fear of angering their nurses, doctors, and schedulers.

Don't let that happen to you. Don't worry if the hospital gets angry; they will get over it. Don't worry if your doctors are inconvenienced; that is their job. Your only concern is that you arrive at the best medical decision possible, even if you change your mind twenty times. After all, medical care is about your good health, not a popularity contest.

Do what's right for you.

NINETEEN

The Good and Bad of Afterward

UNLIKE MOST HOLLYWOOD MOVIES, endings to our medical decisions do not have to be happy. And in real life, even happy endings frequently have problems.

AFTERWARD: WHEN THINGS GO WRONG

Our best decisions can result in sad endings. The treatment we chose for our cancer may fail, leading to more disfiguring treatment or even death. The cosmetic surgery we choose may leave us ugly, the medicine we take may destroy our ability to taste food or make love, and so on. Unlike a movie, however, we cannot simply walk out of the theater into a different life. We are stuck with our unhappy endings.

I think that the most important thing you can do at this point is to have faith in the person you were in the past, while you were making the decision. You cannot change what has happened, but you can realize that you made the best decision that you could, and that you made this decision for yourself lovingly and with great care. You were not stupid; you did a good job. It's just that life all too often brings bad things to people who do the right thing.

What you should *not* do is second-guess yourself. It is natural to think, "If only I had done it differently, if only I had taken more time to read, or talk with Dr. X. instead of Dr. Y.," or some such thing. Don't. You made your best decision and life went the other way. It's not your fault. Really.

But you may nevertheless find yourself believing your bad outcome was a direct result of mistakes that you made in choosing your medical care. Social psychologists have shown that these feelings of self-recrimination are usually unwarranted, based more on the occurrence of a bad outcome than on objective fact. For example, in reviewing what he termed "hindsight bias," Redelmeier cited a study in which physicians were asked to evaluate appropriateness of care, and found that the physicians were more likely to give a poor rating to the medical care if they knew that the outcome was bad. So again, it is not fair to beat yourself up about past decisions, even if they led to poor outcomes.

And of course we must admit that had you made a different decision, you might be worse off. No one knows the future, and no one can predict what might have happened if you had chosen differently. A patient who chose to undergo knee surgery might end up with an infection and even an amputation. But had he not undergone this ill-fated surgery, who's to say that his knee pain wouldn't have caused him to lose control of his car, killing himself and his family? Dwell on this: We cannot second-guess fate.

In fact, bad outcomes arising from our decisions can hold great meaning for us. The woman with progressive cancer might be motivated to start a fund-raising effort to help other patients, or a long and unexpected convalescence may provide an opportunity to meet and inspire others. No one has said this more eloquently than Viktor Frankl, an Austrian psychiatrist who survived four concentration camps during World War II. His descriptions of those merciless and horrific conditions include surprising accounts of people who found meaning in their suffering. Some camp prisoners actually derived spiritual enrichment from these times, becoming generous and kind to their fellow prisoners at dear cost to themselves. One patient described by

Frankl after the war took meaning from his wife's death, because this tragic event spared her the agony of grieving his death in the future.

Suffering and pain are facts of life. We can only choose how to respond and hope to find meaning in these sorrowful realities.

Don't second-guess fate.

AFTERWARD: WHEN THINGS GO RIGHT

If everything goes as planned and the results are what we wanted, everything is great. Then why, you may ask, do I feel off-center? Why at times do I even feel depressed? The results were good; I should be happy, right?

Not necessarily so. Some of the happiest patients in the world should be those who have had surgery to relieve epilepsy. These poor souls are tortured for years by incapacitating seizures that strike unexpectedly at any time, instantly reducing them to an insensate mass of uncontrolled shaking, screaming, and incontinence. They are not allowed to drive a car, and normal employment is rare. They are usually great financial and emotional challenges to their families, and normal social relationships are often impossible. So, when surgery works, when the portion of the brain causing the seizures is removed without harm, you might expect these patients to be happy, thrilled, grateful, and excited about their new life free of seizures.

The surprising truth, however, is that more than a few of these patients are depressed after their successful surgeries. Many cry at odd times during the day and cannot sleep, seemingly unable to enjoy their new life. Although nearly all of them will eventually recover from this depression, they are miserable in the short run.

I believe that the reason patients experience this postoperative depression is that the happy endings delivered by surgery also bring about major changes in self-image and in the viewpoints of others. The direction of their lives and the role they play in the lives around them are dramatically changed by the simple fact that they no longer have seizures. Major changes like these, even good ones, are stressful, and stress provides a fertile breeding ground for depression and anxiety. The relationship between major changes, stress, and depression may not be direct, but we cannot deny that successful surgery is capable of bringing about the stress of major change.

So, be patient with yourself. You have traveled a long road. You have discovered your medical problem, gathered facts, ruminated long and hard, made your decisions, and you now have seen the happy consequences. A major event of your life has transpired, one filled with stress, anxiety, and risk. Give yourself time to adapt to the changes and to catch up on all the events. It is normal to be off-center and even depressed at this point, but with time you will regain your equilibrium and enjoy your fortunate and well-deserved happy outcome.

Happy endings are hard, too.

Part VII
How to Begin

TWENTY

An Example: Cancer

IT BEGINS WITH A SMALL LUMP, almost unannounced except that you find it without looking. Or a mild pain, or a slight shortness of breath. You ignore it for a while, then go to the doctor just to see what it might be. A few tests, one thing leads to another, and then—you can't believe it: you have cancer.

Your doctor explains the diagnosis to you, what it might mean for the future, and what you should do now. He or she will want to schedule more tests, or perhaps a biopsy. Chemotherapy, radiation, and surgery are mentioned. And as the discussion proceeds, you may find that you are not listening at all.

Remember that at this stage, you are not yourself. As we discussed in chapter two, you may feel isolated from others who do not seem to have medical problems, and you may feel disoriented by the magnitude of your problem. You may think that decisions are not necessary, especially if you are overwhelmed by these new circumstances and frightened by the consequences that decisions might bring. Chapter two gives some ways to cope with these feelings, feelings that will become less painful with time.

As you regain some of your equilibrium, it dawns on you that you have some tough decisions to face and much to learn. Remember the points made in our section of general advice (Part I). Remember that you must be hopeful even while realizing there are no guarantees. Remember that *whom* you obtain your medical care from is critical, and that you should assign one of your doctors as your captain. Remember that you will solve your problems in your own style, as you have solved others in the past. And don't forget to take some breaks.

STEP 1: IDENTIFICATION OF YOUR OPTIONS

Your first task, and part of Step 1, will be to decide where you will obtain your medical care. Should you stay with your own doctors, or seek out specialists? What about traveling to prestigious centers? Is there treatment offered elsewhere that is not available locally? These issues are discussed in chapter five. It is also helpful to discuss these questions with your doctors, friends, and family. You may wish to use some of the methods discussed in chapter seven to search the medical literature and the Internet for the expertise available at other centers.

The other part of Step 1 is to identify your options. This will naturally take place as you talk with your doctors and read about your medical condition. How much testing should you undergo to detect other sites of tumor? How often should you be tested? Is your tumor best treated with chemotherapy? Is there a role for surgery to remove the tumor? Is chemotherapy a good idea, and can it be combined with radiation therapy? Are there different types of chemotherapy, and are there different types of radiation? Do you need any treatment at all? Are there different types of experimental protocols available? Is there a role for vaccines, immunotherapy or other methods? It may require some work to find all of your options.

STEP 2: IDENTIFICATION OF TRADEOFFS

Step 2 is to identify the tradeoffs. Again, discussions with your doctors and some research through medical literature will be essential, and we have discussed some ways to pull this together in chapter six. Questions will arise such as: What are the potential complications of chemotherapy? How effective is surgery at prolonging life? Will I be disfigured by surgery? Am I at any risk of losing sexual function? What are the risks of radiation? What are the risks of deferring radiation? What if I do nothing? You need to know the pros and cons of each of the possible medical treatments.

STEP 3. DISCOVERY OF DATA

As you mull over these difficult questions, you will be reading medical articles, searching through the Internet, and talking with your doctors and friends. These activities constitute our Step 3, the discovery of data, and are discussed thoroughly in chapter seven. You may wish to use these methods to read about your tumor in a medicine textbook, then in a surgery textbook, and then in a general textbook about cancer. Remember that you do not have to understand all of the technical details, and that some of the information may be frightening. You may wish to use Web sites such as MEDLINEplus to find articles about your tumor; remember that you can search for review articles to gain a general perspective of your problem. And Web sites such as that of the National Cancer Institute are often good sources of important information.

STEP 4: INTERPRETATION OF NUMBERS

Chapter eight helps you in Step 4, the interpretation of all the information you find in your search. Even if you do not want to get into the details of the statistical analysis of medical testing, it is a good idea to scan this chapter. It will help you build some healthy skepticism and interpret the various conflicting claims you might encounter.

STEP 5: GATHERING YOUR BELIEFS

Behind the scenes, in the back of your mind, your private beliefs and assumptions influence how you think about these medical matters and how you make your medical decisions. Is cancer an inevitable part of your life, just another stage to experience? Or is it an intrusion, something to be fought tooth and nail? What actions can you take to maintain control over your life at this point? Which types of medical information will you believe, and whom do you trust? These important and personal issues are discussed in chapter nine as our Step 5, and should be given the full importance they deserve as you make your decisions.

STEP 6: CONTEMPLATION OF MEANING

Finally, we must consider the meaning that each of our decisions holds for us. How will a life-saving mastectomy affect your self-image and personal life? How well will you cope with a prostatectomy if it results in impotence? Can you live with the threat of tumor recurrence if you do not have these procedures? Is the added safety of chemotherapy worth the risk of prolonged nausea and vomiting? The answers to these questions are rooted in our ideas about the meaning of our existence and our role in the world. Some advice and considerations are given in chapter ten.

In any treatment of cancer, doctors play a crucial role. You will probably see more doctors than you ever knew existed and be subjected to more opinions than you care to hear. Part V of this book shows you how to cope with the different roles and personalities of the doctors you encounter, even when they disagree.

You may be deciding for someone else, or you may have special problems not covered by the six steps. These situations are discussed in Parts VI and VII.

Finally, as time passes and your decisions are made, the results of your treatment will probably be a mixture of events both happy and sad. Remember, as we discussed in chapter eighteen, that there are ways to tell if your decisions are good. And remember from chapter nineteen not to blame yourself for decisions that lead to bad news and to be patient with yourself during the inevitable stress of a happy ending.

Recommended Reading

HERE ARE A FEW BOOKS that I think have important things to say about decisions and the pitfalls of making choices. Most of these do not focus on medical matters, but their insights are valuable for those making medical decisions.

The first three books are treasure troves of practical advice and unexpected insights.

How We Know What Isn't So, by Thomas Gilovich (The Free Press, 1991). Just as its title promises, this book shows us how much of what we firmly believe is in fact utterly false. Gilovich explains why we insist on believing what isn't so, using both medical and nonmedical examples. A must-read for anyone wanting more information about the prejudices that shape everyone's thinking.

The Psychology of Judgment and Decision Making, by Scott Plous (McGraw-Hill, 1993). This delightful, short book explains and illustrates the many fallacies that plague us all when we make decisions. By use of clever examples and lucid text, Plous makes the latest findings from the field of social psychology both understandable and amusing.

Decision Traps. The Ten Barriers to Brilliant Decision-Making and How to Overcome Them, by J. Edward Russo and Paul J.H. Schoemaker (Simon and Schuster, 1990). This useful book was written with business decisions in mind, but is equally applicable for medical decisions. The authors focus on the practical aspects of making decisions, giving a useful list of mistakes and how to avoid them. A good source of practical advice.

The next two books are more theoretical, but offer useful background and viewpoints that will help anyone's search for good medical decisions.

Making Choices. A Recasting of Decision Theory, by Frederic Schick (Cambridge University Press, 1997). This short, academic book approaches decision making from the philosophical viewpoint. What are decisions, how do they fit in with our view of the world, what are the ethical considerations? This book gives a nice theoretical background for approaching decisions.

The Practice of Autonomy. Patients, Doctors and Medical Decisions, by Carl E. Schneider (Oxford University Press, 1998). This is a thoughtful and provocative book, offering the theme that contrary to current ethical dogma, patients would rather their doctor make their medical decisions than themselves. Though not always kind to modern medicine, Schneider's intensive study of patients and decisions is food for thought for anyone wishing to understand our ambivalent relationship with doctors.

Index